THE PROSTATE BOOK

The
PROSTATE
BOOK

Sound Advice on
Symptoms and Treatment

Revised and Updated Edition

STEPHEN N. ROUS, M.D.

Illustrations by Betty Goodwin

W·W·NORTON & COMPANY
New York   London

The text of this book is composed in Baskerville,
with display type set in Fritz Quadrata.
Composition and manufacturing by
The Maple-Vail Book Manufacturing Group.
Book design by Jacques Chazaud.

Library of Congress Cataloging-in-Publication Data
Rous, Stephen N. (Stephen Norman), 1931–
The prostate book : sound advice on symptoms and the treatment /
Stephen Rous.—Updated ed.
p.   cm.
Includes index.
1. Prostate—Diseases—Popular works.   I. Title.
RC899.R672 1992
616.6'5—dc20   91–38775

ISBN 0-393-03387-2

W. W. Norton & Company, Inc.
500 Fifth Avenue, New York, N.Y. 10110
W. W. Norton & Company Ltd.
10 Coptic Street, London WC1A 1 PU

2 3 4 5 6 7 8 9 0

This book,
with much love,
is for
Margot, Ben, and David

Acknowledgments

Writing a book like this is undeniably a good deal of work but it is also really very enjoyable. It is made even more enjoyable by the help and the cooperation of colleagues. In that vein I would like to express my deep appreciation to several of these former colleagues at the Medical University of South Carolina without whose very gracious input this book would have been immeasurably more difficult and time-consuming to complete. Dr. Nancy Curry, our priceless uroradiologist, kindly allowed me to use many, if not all, of the x-rays and CT scans included in this book; Dr. Leonie Gordon, nuclear medicine specialist, supplied me with the various radionuclide scans shown in Chapter 2; and Dr. Ken Spicer kindly allowed me to use his MRI (magnetic resonance imaging) studies of the prostate.

My very closest erstwhile colleagues, those in the Department of Urology at the Medical University, were Drs. William Turner, Robert Nelson, Ian Aaronson, and Nabil Bissada. They were extremely helpful as sounding boards for my ideas and for offering many wonderful suggestions on their own. I do thank them so very much for all of their help and for their patience while I was writing this book—and not doing other things that someone else then had to do!

Betty Goodwin, chief of medical illustrations at the Medical University, was able to turn my not very well expressed thoughts and ideas into beautiful drawings that perfectly illustrated what I had hoped to illustrate. Susan Pullen, my secretary, never lost her cool as she revised this manuscript again and again, and then yet once again. Her many excellent suggestions were gratefully accepted, and I will always appreciate her incredible efficiency and her superb cheerfulness as she labored at her word processor for many, many hours. Would that I could keep her with me forever in all my future endeavors!

Finally, to Mary Cunnane, my editor on this book, I owe a great deal of thanks and appreciation because she taught me, with a gentle firmness, that there is a great deal of difference between writing a book for medical professionals and writing one for the laity.

Contents

Introduction

I am often asked by lay people to describe my specialty of urology. The best answer that I have been able to come up with is that urology is the medical and surgical treatment of diseases of the urinary tract in men, women, and children and the reproductive tract in males. I then sometimes add that these many and varied diseases occur in all age groups, from the newborn to the very aged. Before I can say much more about my favorite subject, I am usually interrupted by a man saying,

"Urology? The urinary tract? The reproductive tract? That must mean that you know all about the prostate too. Listen, I hate to talk shop outside of office hours, but could you just explain why it is that . . ."

The man with the problem was not any different from most men that I have met in thirty years of practicing urology. Without a doubt, the prostate gland seems to generate more questions, more misunderstandings, more concern, and more anxieties than any other part of the male genitourinary tract. This really isn't at all surprising, though, because the prostate gland does indeed cause more grief for more men than just about any other structure in the body, and the symptoms and difficulties arising from the prostate cover almost the entire adult life of a man.

When I was asked by my publisher if I would be willing to write a book about the prostate, I quite literally jumped at the opportunity to do so, because I have found that a major part of practicing the specialty which I love so much is taken up by patients with prostatic problems. At least daily, I find myself explaining to patients why their prostate gland is causing them grief, discussing the rationale for my recommended treatment, whether medical or surgical, and particularly dispelling the many myths and outright falsehoods that patients have learned about the prostate gland. I do not believe that there is any book currently available for the lay reader that covers the subject of prostatic diseases in the manner in which I would like to see it covered. I was therefore happy to write such a book for the benefit of my patients and the patients of my colleagues. Perhaps this book should even have been dedicated to all those men who have ever suffered from any prostatic diseases or perhaps to those men who will yet suffer the misery of this affliction.

If you are reading this book I imagine that you have been told that you have a disease of your prostate gland, or perhaps you think that you may have such a disease, or perhaps you know someone afflicted with one of the maladies of the prostate. In this book I will try to help you to understand your prostate as fully as possible so that you and your doctor will hopefully be able to overcome your problem, handle your problem, or at the very least learn to live with your problem.

There are three distinct and different types of diseases that affect the prostate gland and they occur, for the most part, at different periods of a man's life. Infection and inflammation of the prostate tend to occur at a relatively young age, and most men with this problem are between the ages of 25 and 45. The second of the diseases affecting the prostate is benign prostatic hyperplasia, usually known simply as BPH, which generally begins to produce symptoms at about age 45 or 50. BPH is extremely common and it is probable that most men in the United States who are over the age of 50 have at least some of the symptoms of this condition. The last of the conditions affecting the prostate is cancer, which is very rare before age 50 but which then increases in frequency as a man gets older. Prostate cancer is the most common cancer in American men (excluding skin cancer) and the second most common (to lung cancer) cause of cancer death. In this book

I will discuss each of these three distinct conditions at length so that you will understand fully the symptoms they produce, the various tests that I feel should be used in their diagnosis, and specific forms of therapy which I have found to be most effective in each of these groups of conditions.

I have learned that the prostate gland in many ways is different from other structures of the body that are prone to the same types of diseases. Most men think of the prostate gland as a genital or sexual structure, and I suppose that this is so in the strictest sense of the word since the main function of the prostate is to produce the fluid in which spermatozoa travel to the outside of the body during orgasm and ejaculation. Unfortunately, however, because of this perception of the prostate as a sexual structure, I have found that most men tend to be extraordinarily frightened about prostatic disease of any kind and they are generally much more worried than I might otherwise expect them to be based only on the symptoms themselves. I am constantly amazed at the widespread prevalence of the firm belief that prostatic infection or inflammation, or even BPH, will lead to that most feared of all conditions, the inability to achieve an erection! This one single fear I have found to be of overriding concern to virtually all men. I have found this fear to be partly based upon the dismal prospect of not being able to have sexual intercourse, but I have also found that to most men the potential to perform intercourse is just as important as the act itself because these men feel that they cannot possibly be true men if they cannot perform sexually.

If there is anything that I have learned from my patients in thirty years it is that treating their physical ailments is simply not sufficient when these ailments are prostatic in origin. Whatever extra time is required to put the disease in perspective for my patients, to explain exactly what the disease is, and particularly to reiterate time and again that these prostatic problems are not related to the ability to perform sexually, has all been time extremely well spent. It has been estimated that about half of all the complaints bringing patients to primary care physicians are psychosomatic in origin. While I do not believe this figure to be nearly that high with urological problems presented to a urologist, I am totally and absolutely convinced of the necessity of recognizing the mental anguish and outright fear of many of my patients and in taking whatever time is necessary to address these concerns, to allay the fears, and to reassure my patients that their dreaded concerns will not materialize.

Because diseases of the prostate gland are so very widespread and prevalent, I have found that most of them are initially treated by a primary care physician. This is often perfectly satisfactory initially and in cases where a patient responds rapidly to therapy. However, for those patients with infection or inflammation that does not improve, for those patients with BPH, and particularly for those patients with prostatic cancer, I feel that the only acceptable form of therapy is that given by a urologist.

Since that statement is a very strong one, I feel that I should tell you why I have said it. Only a urologist has had the extensive and excellent training required to care for these complex urologic diseases. The training of the urologist is a long and arduous one extending for five and very often six years following graduation from medical school. This training is carried out in one of approximately 120 approved programs in the United States and it invariably is in a highly specialized university medical center. During the course of these five or six years, the embryo urologist, who is known as a urology resident, is exposed to the entire spectrum of urologic diseases. He or she is taught urologic diagnosis and treatment by professors of urology in these university medical centers, many of whom are truly distinguished educators and clinicians. The educational process of the urology resident is a step-by-step one culminating in the final year of training in which the resident is responsible for the medical and surgical treatment of large numbers of patients, always under the supervision of a university faculty member.

At the completion of the last year of residency training, known as the chief resident year, the embryo urologist (who is now 31 or 32 years of age) sits for an all-day written examination that is given by the American Board of Urology and that covers all of the aspects of urology that have been studied during the previous five or six years. After completing the residency, the new urologist is now permitted to practice urology in a community of his choosing where he is constantly and carefully monitored by other urologic colleagues in the community and by the senior urologist at the hospital in which patient care is delivered.

Assuming that the new urologist practices competent urology as determined by a group of peers in the same community, he or she is then allowed to take the oral examinations of the American Board of Urology which are given approximately eighteen months after the written examinations have been taken and passed. The oral exams are administered by at least two very senior academic urologists who are invariably professors of urology in their own universities. This oral portion of the examination includes a demonstration of competence in x-ray interpretation and recognition of the microscopic appearance of surgical specimens. Satisfactory completion of this second part of the examination entitles the new urologist to be a Diplomate of the American Board of Urology. Receipt of this prestigious and coveted certificate means that the individual physician can then truly be considered an expert and a specialist in urologic diseases. There are only about 9,000 practicing physicians in the United States who have earned this privilege.

Urology, like virtually all other branches of medicine, is an art as well as a science. This means, among other things, that the treatment of patients is not necessarily a set thing, where A will always follow B as it would in a pure science. There are often many treatment options for the same disease because no one treatment exists that works 100 percent of the time. Similarly, even the diagnostic steps taken in determining why a patient has such and such symptoms are not always cut and dried and are not always the same steps that would be taken in the same situation by every other physician.

Different physicians who are equally bright and equally capable will follow different diagnostic routes to the same end and will use different methods of treating the same disease. Neither physician is necessarily wrong, for the differences reflect the fact that in the hands of a given physician one treatment has consistently shown better results than another, and physicians will have differing experiences that will lead to different conclusions.

Throughout this book, I frequently have expressed my own opinions about the diagnosis and treatment of many urologic problems. However, my opinions are just that and certainly are not meant in any way to imply that others who may differ with me are wrong.

Finally, I hope that this book will fulfill the expectations of my readers; I will be satisfied if this book serves to comfort and to reassure those men suffering from the various diseases of the prostate.

THE PROSTATE BOOK

1

Normal Anatomy and Normal Function

I have always found the study of anatomy to be tedious. It involves rote memory work without the necessity of thinking very much. I have also come to realize that an intimate knowledge of anatomy is not at all necessary for internists or family physicians, but it really *is* very important for surgeons who must make daily use of this knowledge.

I also believe that some very basic knowledge of the anatomy and the normal function of the prostate will help you to better understand any difficulty that you may be having and its treatment.

The normal prostate gland in the adult male lies between the urinary bladder and the external urethral sphincter, the muscle that a man tightens when he wants to shut off his flow of urine (Fig. 1–1). The adult prostate gland is about the size and shape of a large chestnut and it weighs about 20 grams, or a little less than one ounce. At the time of birth, the prostate is about the size of a pea. It gradually increases in size until puberty, when there is a period of rapid growth that continues until the third decade of life, when the prostate reaches its normal adult size. The size of the prostate gland

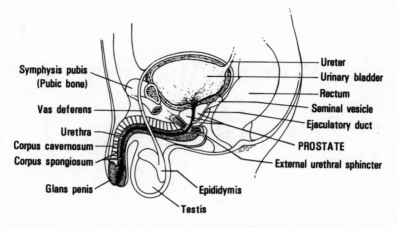

Symphysis pubis
(Pubic bone)

Vas deferens

Urethra

Corpus cavernosum

Corpus spongiosum

Glans penis

Epididymis

Testis

Ureter

Urinary bladder

Rectum

Seminal vesicle

Ejaculatory duct

PROSTATE

External urethral sphincter

Figure 1–1   *The entire male genitourinary tract. This figure shows the relationship of the prostate gland to the urinary bladder and the external urethral sphincter. It also illustrates the other genitourinary tract structures. This is a lateral view taken through the precise midpoint of the male body.*

then remains constant until about age 40 or 45, at which time benign prostatic hyperplasia (BPH) commences in most men. BPH is a process of aging in which the prostate gland enlarges by a multiplication of its cells and which is usually, but not always, accompanied by symptoms of difficulty voiding. This growth will continue very slowly until death. In a relatively few very fortunate men, BPH just does not develop; these men will never have any of the symptoms commonly associated with this condition. In these very few and lucky men the prostate slowly decreases in size over the remaining years of life, a condition that is normal for these men.

The anatomic fact that I have found most confusing to patients and even to some physicians may also be confusing to you. I refer to the relationship of the prostate gland to the prostatic urethra, of the prostatic urethra to the rest of the urethra, and of the prostate gland to the bladder. The way that I have found best to simplify this is to ask you to think of

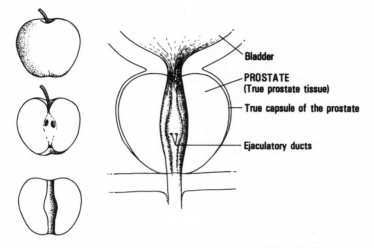

Figure 1–2   *The prostate gland. This shows the prostate looking like an apple which has been cut in half with the core removed.*

the prostate gland as an apple with the core removed (Fig. 1–2). The prostatic urethra is then that portion of the urethra which is within the prostate gland and has precisely the same anatomic relationship to the gland as the core of the apple has to the apple itself. The entire urethra is a channel through which urine flows when it leaves the bladder; the prostatic urethra is the first part of that channel (Fig. 1–3). The prostatic urethra ends at the external urethral sphincter. It is the sphincter muscle which you voluntarily contract when you want to suddenly stop your flow of urine while voiding. The very small portion of the urethra that passes through the external sphincter muscle is known as the membranous urethra. The next part of the urethra going from the bladder to the penis is known as the bulbous urethra. The last and often the longest portion of the urethra is external and is known as the penile or the pendulous urethra. You will note that the internal portion of the urethra may at times be almost as long as the external portion. To say it once again, the prostatic urethra is

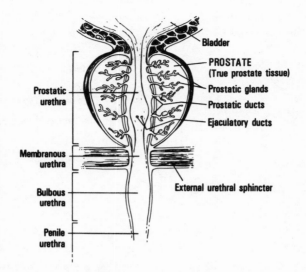

Figure 1–3   *The relationship of the prostate gland to the prostatic ure-thra and to each of the other portions of the urethra.*

nothing more than a straight channel through the prostate gland through which urine flows as soon as it leaves the bladder.

If you were to look at your prostate under a microscope you would see that it is composed of muscle, glands, and fibrous or connective tissue. These same types of tissue comprise benign prostatic hyperplasia (BPH) when it arises. The only difference between the normal prostate tissue and the BPH tissue is that the latter generally has more muscle and fibrous tissue than the normal prostate.

There are many, many small glands within the prostate, and each of these pour their secretions into one of the prostatic ducts during orgasm and ejaculation. These ducts in turn empty into the prostatic urethra. The ducts that carry the spermatozoa also empty into the prostatic urethra; these are called the ejaculatory ducts. These ducts, in addition to bringing the spermatozoa into the prostatic urethra, also bring fluid from the seminal vesicles which are sac-like structures, two in number, directly behind the base of the bladder. The seminal vesicles provide some of the fluid that serves as a nutrient for the spermatozoa. The vast majority of the sperm reach the ejaculatory ducts via the vas deferens which are paired, cord-like structures through which the sperm are transported from the testis and epididymis. It is these vas deferens structures that are surgically divided during the very popular contraceptive operation known as a vasectomy. During orgasm, spermatozoa, fluid from the seminal vesicles, and fluid from the prostate gland all pour into the prostatic urethra because of contractions of the muscles of the prostate and the seminal vesicles. This mixture of fluids is then propelled to the outside during ejaculation by the spasmodic contractions of the muscles that surround the urethra.

The prostate is referred to as an accessory sex gland. It is considered to be an accessory (and not a primary) part of the sexual or reproductive tract because, even though its sole function is sexual, it is only indirectly involved in procreation. Obviously, the testes are the site of the manufacture of spermatozoa, and the penis is necessary to deliver the spermatozoa into the upper reaches of the vagina. The testes and the penis are therefore considered to be the primary sexual structures. The prostate is considered to be a gland because it makes secretions and thereby meets the definition of a gland. These secretions are manufactured within the prostatic glands and enter the prostatic urethra, along with fluid from the ejaculatory ducts, at the time of orgasm and ejaculation (Fig. 1–4). All of these secretions then go to the outside of the body during ejaculation and so the prostate is known as an externally secreting gland. In contrast, the male body has endocrine glands such as the testis, the adrenal, and the pituitary, all of which produce internal secretions that go throughout the body via the bloodstream.

The principal function of the prostate gland is to produce the fluid that comprises the vast majority of the semen. The primary purpose of this fluid is to serve as a vehicle in which

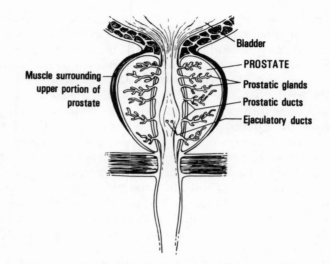

Bladder

PROSTATE

Muscle surrounding
upper portion of
prostate

Prostatic glands

Prostatic ducts

Ejaculatory ducts

Figure 1–4   *The prostate gland, showing the numerous glands within the prostate and the relationship of these glands to the prostatic ducts. Note the presence of the ejaculatory ducts which empty into the prostatic urethra from the vas deferens and the seminal vesicles.*

the spermatozoa can travel to the outside at the time of ejaculation. Prostatic fluid secondarily provides some nourishment to the spermatozoa.

An understanding of the male reproductive system will be helpful to you so that you can better place the role of the prostate in its proper perspective (Fig. 1–5). Each testis is located in the scrotum and has two principal functions, both of which are controlled by hormones from the pituitary gland. First, the testis manufactures the spermatozoa needed for procreation. This is done in very small tubules within the testis known as seminiferous tubules. The testis also manufactures almost all of the body's principal male hormone, testosterone. This is produced by the Leydig cells which are also within the testis. These cells discharge the testosterone directly into the bloodstream. For this reason the testis is considered to be an endocrine gland. The spermatozoa which are manufactured in the testis converge into a network of ducts

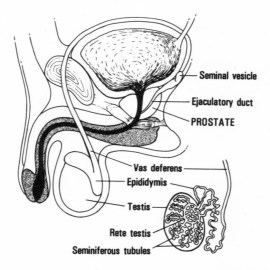

Figure 1–5 *The male reproductive system, showing details of the testis and the relationship of the testis to the epididymis, to the vas deferens, to the seminal vesicle, and to the ejaculatory duct.*

which then lead into the epididymis, a structure which is just behind the testis and connected to it by means of a network of ducts (the rete testis). The epididymis is a long, coiled tubular structure which provides a storage place for the spermatozoa to mature and then go on their way when needed. The vas deferens is a paired small and heavily muscled tubular structure which conveys the spermatozoa from the epididymis to the seminal vesicles and ejaculatory ducts. These in turn empty into the prostatic urethra at the time of orgasm and ejaculation. The muscles of the vas deferens serve to propel the spermatozoa in their journey towards the prostatic urethra. The seminal vesicle itself is a paired structure that is really little more than a storage sac located behind the base of the bladder. It manufactures and stores a nutrient fluid for the spermatozoa to use during their journey through the urethra, into a woman's vagina, uterus, and up into the fallopian tubes in order to fertilize an ovum. Occasionally, spermatozoa may be stored within the seminal vesicle; how much of this occurs is really a function of the frequency of ejaculation.

During sexual stimulation the penis becomes erect because of an increased flow of blood into the paired, spongy bodies (corpora cavernosa) which lie within the penis. At the height of sexual excitement, orgasm takes place, a phenomenon produced by muscular contractions which propel spermatozoa and fluid from the prostate and seminal vesicles into the prostatic urethra and then to the outside of the body, known as ejaculation. The strong muscles which surround the prostate and urethra propel the ejaculate to the outside, while at the same time the bladder neck closes to prevent the ejaculated fluid from going back into the bladder. Of the total amount of fluid in the ejaculate, something under 5 percent contains spermatozoa; the remainder is made up of fluid from the prostate gland and to a much lesser degree fluid from the seminal vesicles. A very small component of the ejaculate is fluid from the small glands that surround the urethra. The prostate makes and stores its secretions more or less continuously and for all practical purposes these secretions are never totally emptied from the prostate. The production of fluid will vary with the demand, which in turn is a function of the frequency of ejaculation and the status of the fluid within the prostate at any given time.

2

How the Doctor Diagnoses Your Problems

From the earliest days of medical school we doctors have been told to "listen to the patient if you want to know what's wrong with him." I agree with this completely, and I have found that I can usually form an accurate impression of my patient's problem simply by listening to him relate his symptoms and by then knowing which questions to ask in order to home in on a tentative diagnosis. This process is known as "taking a history" from a patient.

I next examine my patient, placing particular emphasis on those details of the physical examination which I think will yield the most information, based upon the history that I have already received. As it usually turns out, the combination of a well-taken history and a good physical examination of the genitourinary tract are sufficient for me to reach a provisional diagnosis of the cause of my patient's problem. For most patients, though, what I *think* is the cause of their problem is not sufficient; they want me to be absolutely certain of the diagnosis that I give to them.

Diagnosing with precision the various disorders of the prostate can be a tricky business, but we urologists happily have at our disposal a large variety of excellent diagnostic tests that we can administer. From these many tests, though, only a selected few are chosen, and I will always try to choose the *fewest* possible number of studies needed in order to be absolutely certain of my diagnosis. I look upon those diagnostic studies that I do obtain as very necessary in order to confirm the provisional diagnosis that I have made from the history and physical exam. Occasionally, though, the diagnostic studies serve to refute my provisional diagnosis and force me to rethink it.

I fully recognize that you, as a patient, may have considerable dismay about the various tests that we urologists do. This is not only because of the natural aversion that many people have to physicians and their tests but because of the very intimate area of the body with which we urologists deal. I assure you that we do the absolute minimum number of studies compatible with reaching a correct diagnosis, and I further assure you that virtually all of the studies done by urologists are far more unpleasant to contemplate than they are to undergo! Discussed below are several of the most frequently done diagnostic studies, but always remember that you will most likely need to have only a very few of these.

Examination of the Urine

This single test probably provides more information about a patient and his genitourinary tract per dollar of cost than any other. It is really a screening test since it alone does not provide any definitive diagnoses but serves as a red flag alerting a physician to look further. Although a urine analysis is able to detect sugar in the urine of diabetic patients, the part of the urinalysis that is directly related to prostatic diseases is the microscopic examination and the culture of the urine. The microscopic part of the urine examination is helpful in a patient with prostatic disease since it will show white blood cells (pus cells) which may possibly be indicative of infection. It can also demonstrate the presence of red blood cells which may be due to an insignificant problem, such as a mild inflammation in the urethra or bladder, or it may indicate a life-threatening tumor. Anything over 0–2 red blood cells per high power microscopic field is generally considered to be abnormal, although not necessarily serious.

A culture of the urine is absolutely necessary if infection in the urinary tract is to be diagnosed with any certainty. Any microscopic exam of the urine showing more than 1–3 white blood cells per high power field is generally considered to be abnormal, although not necessarily indicative of any disease. The presence of these white blood cells should suggest at least the possibility of infection in the urinary tract and I feel that it is incorrect to make a definite diagnosis of infection without culturing the urine.

A urine culture is obtained from the middle portion of the urinary stream, after a man retracts his foreskin and cleans the glans penis well with soap and water. A circumcised man does not need to do this cleaning procedure. Midstream urine is obtained by having a man start to void the first few ounces of urine into the toilet, then collect the middle portion of his stream in a sterile container, and then finish emptying his bladder directly into the toilet. At no point in this process should the urinary stream be stopped or interrupted. One milliliter of the urine obtained from the middle portion of the urinary stream is then transferred to a small dish which contains a nutrient on which bacteria (if present) will grow when placed in an incubator at a temperature that is suitable for bacterial growth. After 24 hours of incubation, any bacteria present in the urine can be identified by its growth pattern in the dish, and the number of bacteria present per milliliter of urine can actually be counted. At the same time as the cultures are being done, small cardboard-like disks, impregnated with various antibiotics, are placed in a section of the dish to see which antibiotics are effective against any bacteria that may be growing. It usually takes about a day for a urine culture and bacterial sensitivity study to be done. This study should always be done before a diagnosis of an infection is made, even though an infection may be suspected from the presence of white blood cells in the urine.

Blood Tests to See How Well
the Kidneys Are Working

Two of the blood tests that are commonly used to measure kidney function are known as urea nitrogen and creatinine. When the kidneys are functioning normally these tests have normal values, but when there is diminished kidney function the blood levels of urea nitrogen and creatinine will often rise to abnormal levels. Urea is formed normally in the liver from the breakdown of protein, and it is then found in the blood as urea nitrogen or blood urea nitrogen (BUN), as it is more commonly known. Normally, most of the urea nitrogen is excreted in the urine; its level in the blood will be abnormally high if the kidneys are not working well enough to excrete it in normal amounts. The urea nitrogen levels can also be raised or lowered by abnormalities within the body that have nothing whatever to do with kidney function. For example, since urea is formed within the liver, it can be depressed to extremely low levels if a patient suffers from liver failure and is therefore not able to manufacture urea. Such might be the case even if the kidney function were also severely diminished. However, the creatinine level in the blood is generally not dependent on any bodily functions other than kidney function. For these reasons, then, the creatinine level in the blood is a much more accurate measurement of kidney function than is the urea nitrogen level. Creatinine is produced from the normal breakdown of body muscle; this is the reason that a heavily muscled man will have a higher normal creatinine level than a very small man with minimal muscle mass. All of the creatinine that is made is removed from the blood by the kidneys and excreted into the urine.

Abnormal elevations of the creatinine (and the urea nitrogen as well) generally *do* indicate a decrease in kidney function, but this is not necessarily irreversible or permanent. For example, if there is obstruction to the drainage of urine from both kidneys—as there might well be from a very large prostate gland that is preventing the bladder from emptying—the blood creatinine level might be elevated because the kidneys cannot function normally in the face of the obstruction. Once the blockage of the kidneys is relieved, the blood creatinine level may well return to normal. Whether or not it does so is based on how normal the kidneys were before the obstruction occurred and how long the obstruction was present. It should be noted, relative to the blood creatinine level, that if only one-half of one kidney is functioning normally, the blood creatinine level will still be in the normal range. In other words, the human body has a great deal of reserve renal function.

Normal creatinine levels vary with age and muscle mass, but in the adult male the level is generally between 1.2 and 1.5 mg/100 ml of blood. This may be somewhat lower in very small men and it normally rises slightly in men over age 60.

Blood Tests to Determine the Presence of Prostate Cancer

Prostatic fraction of serum acid phosphatase and prostate specific antigen (PSA) are blood tests of major importance. The prostatic fraction of serum acid phosphatase is made by the normal cells within the prostate gland, but it is also made in equal amounts by any malignant cells that may be within the prostate gland. Malignant prostate cells may "break out" of the prostate gland and appear in other places around the body where they continue to make acid phosphatase, thus elevating its value above the normal level. This is the role of the blood acid phosphatase level; its values are usually normal when there is no cancer of the prostate or when there is cancer confined to the prostate gland. Its values are elevated when prostatic cancer cells are spread outside of the prostate gland.

Although this test is usually accurate, its sensitivity is such that false negatives do exist about 20 percent of the time; that is, normal values are reported when they should be elevated. False positives may also occur, but this is very rare; an elevated acid phosphatase level usually means that the prostate cancer has spread. It is extremely important to stress, however, that prostatic acid phosphatase is manufactured by normal prostatic cells as well as malignant cells; therefore it *cannot* be used as a screening test to detect early prostatic cancer that is still confined within the prostate gland itself.

A relatively new blood test called the serum prostate specific antigen (PSA) has largely supplanted the serum prostatic acid phosphatase (PAP) in the determination of the presence and the extent of prostate cancer. Despite the word "specific" in its name, the PSA test is not specific for prostate cancer. "Specific" relates to its production by prostate cells only. Elevation in PSA can occur with BPH (benign prostate hyperplasia—nonmalignant enlargement) of the prostate common to most men over the age of 50 years) and with prostatitis (an acute and sometimes chronic inflammation or infection of the prostate).

Elevations in PSA, especially mild elevations, have to be interpreted with caution in the presence of prostatic enlargement. In general, the higher the PSA value, the more likely the probability of prostate cancer. But even small increases in this protein require careful evaluation by a urologist. In addition, a small number of false negatives are also possible since occasional prostate cancers do not produce enough PSA to produce an abnormal PSA number. As with any medical test, interpretation and follow-up by a qualified physician are necessary. There are on-going attempts to further refine the PSA test so as to differentiate the PSA that is elevated from BPH from the PSA that is elevated from prostate cancer. Thus far, any such differentiation is not possible.

I feel that I should say considerably more about prostate specific antigen (PSA) because it has become an extraordinarily commonly used blood test and it is one which you should understand. This test measures a substance made by the prostate—both the normal prostate and the malignant prostate. However, the cancerous (malignant) prostate makes about ten times as much of this substance as does the benign prostate on a gram-for-gram basis. PSA is most often measured by a technique that uses up to 4.0 ng / ml as the upper limit of normal. If you have a blood PSA level above 4.0 ng / ml it does not necessarily mean that you have cancer of the prostate. If you have a large prostate your blood PSA can be elevated because PSA is made by benign prostate cells as well as malignant ones. If you have had infection in your prostate, your PSA number can be elevated. If your elevation is between 4 and 10, there is only about a 20 percent chance of cancer being present in your prostate—even then it does not mean that the cancer has spread outside of your prostate. As the PSA value goes higher than 10, so do the chances that you have prostate cancer.

It is also important for you to realize that a normal PSA value of under 4.0 ng / ml does not guarantee that you do not have cancer. Indeed, a small cancer might not make enough PSA to get the number over 4.0; worse still, a very malignant cancer might be so primitive in form that it is unable to make any PSA. That situation, fortunately, is uncommon. The important thing for you to realize is that PSA is simply a test that should help your urologist decide what needs to be done next. My own guiding rules, which are simply guides and not written in stone, are that if a patient has a normal digital rectal exam (DRE) of the prostate and his PSA is less than 4.0 ng / ml, I suggest that he return yearly for a DRE and a PSA. If the DRE is abnormal and the PSA is under 4.0, I suggest an ultrasound exam of the prostate with biopsies of the areas that felt abnormal as well as any others that appear abnormal on ultrasound. If the DRE is normal but the PSA is over 4.0 ng / ml I may vary in my management of the case between immediate ultrasound with biopsies and repeating the PSA in three months' time to see if it is rising or stable before deciding on the ultrasound and biopsies.

If the DRE is abnormal and the PSA is over 4.0 ng / ml I will do an ultrasound with biopsies of any suspicious areas or perform random biopsies if no suspicious areas are seen.

Although the PSA test is not considered a "screening" test (indeed, Medicare will only pay for it for those patients already diagnosed with prostate cancer), I still feel it is a wise thing to do in men over 50 years of age or in younger men (over age 40) with a family history of prostate cancer occurring at a young age (prior to age 55). However, I must state emphatically that there is as yet no evidence that diagnosing cancer of the prostate at an early stage affects patient survival, although intuitively one would think it should! The reason is that cancer of the prostate is a two-headed beast which pursues a seemingly benign course in some but not in others. This results in the bottom line that the great majority of men that have prostate cancer die with it and not from it. The problem, of course, is that we don't know which patients will fall into which group!

Finally, a word about the higher PSA numbers. Do we know for sure that very high PSA levels mean the cancer has spread outside of the prostate? The answer is no, and PSA values of 30, 40, and 50 have been noted in which the cancer is still confined within the prostate. However, it is probably safe to say that when the PSA values approach 100 ng / ml it is highly likely that the cancer is no longer confined within the prostate. The levels of PSA fall virtually to zero after the prostate gland is removed in its entirety, as is done with radical prostatectomy. In the years that follow such curative surgery the PSA level is carefully monitored. Should it start to rise it is pretty certain evidence that the cancer has recurred somewhere in the body.

X-ray Studies and Other Imaging Techniques

The Excretory Urogram

Sometimes referred to as an IVP, or intravenous pyelogram, this single x-ray study provides the urologist with an extraordinary amount of information about virtually the entire urinary tract. It is performed by injecting into a vein on the forearm a substance that will concentrate in the kidney and will appear white against the dark background of the x-ray. The white color of the substance within the kidney produces an image on the x-ray film of the kidneys and their interior and then, sequentially, the ureters, the bladder, and the urethra as the injected substance, mixed with urine, moves in a downward fashion from the kidneys towards the bladder and then to the outside. Unfortunately, the substance that is injected in order to perform the x-ray study occasionally causes serious allergic-type reactions and can even cause death, with a reported incidence of fatal reactions between one in 20,000 and one in 80,000 excretory urograms. It is equally unfortunate that it is virtually impossible to predict which individuals will have severe or even fatal reactions to the injected material. Certainly, there is virtually nothing in a person's past history which could make the doctor suspicious of an impending problem, with the possible exception of a known allergy to iodine and iodine products. This is so because iodine is the base for many of these injectable materials. A prior history of a rash or even nausea or vomiting when an excretory urogram has been done is certainly not an indicator that a serious reaction might occur the next time; and a test injection of a small amount of the contrast material is of no benefit either. Certainly a previous excretory urogram that produced a severe fall in blood pressure, an inability to breathe, or some shock-like condition would be a good reason not to do another such study. In patients in whom there is a question about a prior allergic history to the material, a day or two of oral steroids (cortisone) and antihistamines are administered prior to making the x-rays, but whether this offers any real protection against a severe reaction is questionable. A study done not too long ago suggested that one of the major risk factors for a severe reaction following the injection of the contrast material was patient fear and anxiety; so I feel it is very important, should the patient be apprehensive, that everything be done to calm and to reassure him. If this is not possible, it might be advisable to defer the x-ray study. It should go without saying that an excretory urogram because of its inherent, albeit very slight, risk should only be done when there is a true indication for it (see below).

More recently, a new type of injectable substance has been developed which is now widely used and which does not have nearly as great a potential for causing any of these serious or fatal reactions. The cost of this new material, however, is ten or twenty times the cost of the conventional injectable substance, and its use initially has been limited primarily to those individuals felt to be at high risk for an allergic-type reaction. However, it is gradually being used more and more and may well become the standard agent in the near future.

The excretory urogram, which is really a series of films that are exposed over a period of about thirty minutes, is useful for many urologic conditions, but it is primarily used to visualize and examine the kidneys (Fig. 2–1). Its specific rel-

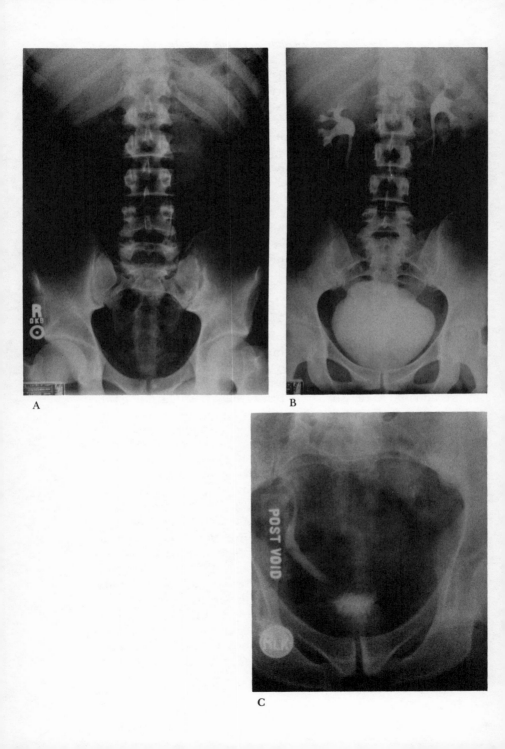

evance to diseases of the prostate gland is therefore somewhat limited. For benign prostatic hyperplasia, the condition that usually accompanies the aging process in men and that makes voiding difficult, the excretory urogram is helpful to estimate how well a patient does or does not empty his bladder during voiding, to see if there is any obstruction to the drainage of the kidneys caused by the enlarged prostate gland, and to get an idea about how large the prostate gland may be by the negative shadow it casts within the bladder itself. The excretory urogram is also used as a broad type of screening test prior to prostate surgery just to make sure that the kidneys have a normal appearance—although it must be noted that many very capable urologists do not feel it necessary to perform this study when surgery on the prostate for BPH is to be undertaken. I feel that the only absolute reason for obtaining an excretory urogram in a patient with BPH is for those patients with microscopic or visible blood in the urine. This is because an excretory urogram is the only totally satisfactory way of making certain that there are no other diseases, such as cancer, in the kidneys and ureters which might be responsible for the blood. In patients with BPH who do not have blood in the urine, I feel that a combination of renal scans and ultrasound (see below) are able to give me all the information I need about a patient's kidneys prior to surgery.

For patients with known prostate cancer, an excretory urogram may be used to demonstrate obstruction to one or

Figure 2–1   *A. KUB film (kidney, ureter, bladder). This is the preliminary film that is taken before any dye is injected into the patient. It shows the kidney areas, the soft tissue areas through which the ureters travel on their way to the bladder, the bladder area, and all of the bony structures.*

B. X-ray taken some minutes after the injection of the dye showing normal kidneys, ureters, and bladder. Note particularly the appearance of the normal and full bladder.

C. A post-void film showing an insignificant amount of dye left in the bladder (arrow). This film is taken after the patient is asked to void the urine and dye that had accumulated in the bladder and that are seen in panel B. Following voiding, there should be an insignificant amount of dye remaining in the bladder.

both kidneys that may occur from a spread of the cancer. This knowledge can be gained equally well from a renal scan. The initial film of the excretory urogram (Fig. 2–1A) can also reveal a cancer spread to one or more of the bones of the pelvis or spine.

For most patients with infection or inflammation of the prostate gland an excretory urogram is not necessary.

Renal Scans

Renal scanning is yet another method of "visualizing" the urinary tract, but the visualization is done by detecting the radioactivity over the kidneys (using a gamma camera) that results when a radioactive material is injected intravenously. This radioactivity is then seen on a monitor and transferred to a piece of paper rather than an x-ray film (Fig. 2–2). The radiation exposure from these renal scans comes from a radioactive material that is injected, but the total amount of radiation is much less than that received by the patient when an excretory urogram (IVP) is done since the radiation exposure to the patient having the IVP procedure is from the x-rays themselves. Furthermore, there is no risk of an allergic-type reaction with a renal scan. The study is particularly suited for those patients with less than normal kidney function because the visualization of poorly functioning kidneys when excretory urograms are done is not very satisfactory. When renal scans are done it is not possible to see the precise anatomic detail within the kidney that is expected from an excretory urogram, but renal scanning is an excellent technique for evaluating the blood flow to the kidneys, how well the kidneys are functioning, and whether there is any obstruction to drainage of the kidneys. Different radioisotopes are concentrated by different parts of the kidney. The isotopes emit gamma rays which are detected by a gamma camera and put on film. These emitted gamma rays will have a characteristic pattern that will depend upon the specific isotope used and therefore the specific cells of the kidney actually concentrating the isotope. The specific pattern of emitted gamma rays for a given individual can then be compared with known nor-

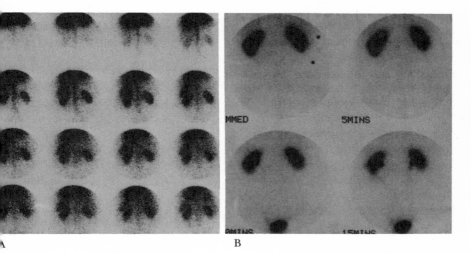

A

B

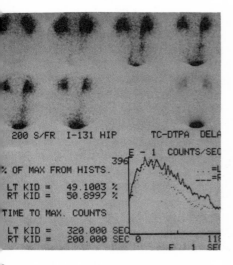

200 S/FR   I-131 HIP

% OF MAX FROM HISTS.

LT KID =   49.1003 %
RT KID =   50.8997 %

TIME TO MAX. COUNTS

LT KID =   320.000 SEC
RT KID =   200.000 SEC

TC-DTPA DELA
E - 1 COUNTS/SEC

C

Figure 2–2   A NORMAL "TRIPLE" RENAL
SCAN.

*A. The blood flow to the kidneys beginning
seconds after the injection of the radioisotope,
and each kidney is seen with equal intensity
showing equal blood flow to the two kidneys.*

*B. Two equal, well-functioning kidneys
several minutes after injection of the radioisotope. The specific kidney function being measured is the glomerular filtration rate, and it
is measured by noting how many minutes it
takes following injection of the radioisotope
for the radioactivity over the kidneys to reach
a maximum.*

*C. Measuring the second major function of
the kidney, known as tubular secretion. This
same image also notes the presence or absence
of any obstruction to the drainage of the kidneys.*

mal patterns for that isotope, thereby permitting the interpretation of renal scans as being normal or abnormal. The use of renal scanning in prostatic diseases is less than that of excretory urography but it probably could be used much more frequently as an alternative diagnostic study to evaluate the kidneys.

Ultrasound

This is a totally noninvasive and benign procedure for which there are literally no risks and no radiation exposure. The procedure is used to image many different structures within the body. When combined with renal scanning it provides virtually as much information about the kidneys (Fig. 2–3) as

Figure 2–3   *Normal ultrasound of the kidney. Arrows outline the kidney. The dark outline in the center of the kidney is caused by the normal complex structures that are in the center of the kidney.*

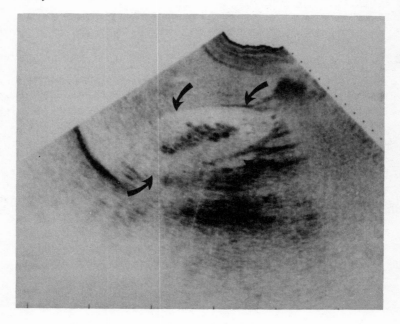

does an excretory urogram, and it is remarkably adept at determining whether various masses found within the kidney on the excretory urograms, for example, are cysts or solid tumors. The principle of ultrasonography is similar to that of sonar which is a means by which objects underwater (as, for example, a submarine) may be identified by a ship on the surface of the water. A series of high-frequency sound waves are generated by the vibration of a crystal within the ultrasound machine, and the crystal then "listens" for the echo response. These responses are transmitted as electrical signals to a screen that records and diagrams these signals, and the shape seen on the screen will reflect the shape and consistency of the object returning the sound waves. Ultrasound in urology is of great use in examining the kidneys and in discriminating between the different types of masses that occur commonly in kidneys, particularly in the differentiation between a mass that is totally cystic (filled with a clear fluid and perfectly benign), one that is solid (with a good possibility of being cancer), and one that is both cystic and solid (which may or may not have cancer within it).

In prostatic diseases, ultrasound has become a major diagnostic tool in determining the presence or absence of prostate cancer. Most urologists feel that ultrasound has a definite role in diagnosing very early prostatic cancer. Moreover, ultrasound is unquestionably of help in visualizing those prostatic cancers that have spread beyond the confines of the prostate gland; the extent of this spread can be nicely visualized on the ultrasound screen. What is still open to question, however, is the role of ultrasound in the *screening* of patients for prostate cancer; most urologists feel that ultrasound is *not* best used in this manner. It is, however, ideally used in a maximizing the accuracy of prostate biopsies in the patient with an abnormal digital rectal exam of the prostate or with an elevated PSA blood test.

For benign prostatic hyperplasia ultrasound can be helpful in estimating the size of the prostate gland in order to determine the best surgical approach to it, since the approach may sometimes be determined by the size of the gland. However, there are certainly equally good methods of estimating size that do not require ultrasound. And, finally, ultrasound adds nothing to the sometimes difficult question of *whether* surgery for BPH is indicated (see Chapter 4).

For prostate infection and inflammation ultrasound would only be of minimal benefit in making a diagnosis, something that could be done correctly and accurately using simpler means (see Chapter 3).

The imaging studies that have just been described—excretory urograms, renal scans, and ultrasound—are sometimes done by urologists and sometimes by radiologists. In the majority of clinical settings in this country, radiologists do the excretory urograms, although a significant number of these studies are done by urologists. The renal scans are mostly done by specialists in nuclear medicine, which is a division of radiology, but a sizable number of urologists also perform them. Ultrasound is probably done for the most part by radiologists at this time, but I feel it will be done increasingly by urologists as an office procedure because there is no radiation risk and no radioactive material involved.

Computed Tomography (CT) Scanning

This extraordinary diagnostic tool has been in common use only since the late 1970s. It is an imaging method that combines the use of x-ray with computer technology. The computer is able to construct a two-dimensional image of a cross section of the body from data obtained by taking x-rays at 1 cm intervals through the part of the body that is being studied. A major advantage of this cross-sectional viewing of the body is in being able to see anatomic, and particularly abnormal, findings in an anterior-posterior relationship that would simply not be seen with standard or conventional x-ray techniques. Besides providing this cross-sectional view (standard x-rays offer a longitudinal view), perhaps the greatest advantage of CT scanning over conventional radiography is the ability of these scans to detect differences in density between parts of the body far better than can be done with more conventional x-ray studies. CT scanning is therefore extraordinarily useful in the evaluation of abnormal masses anywhere in the body because the scans are able to determine whether or not these masses are dense enough to be a malignant tumor or are, in fact, benign masses. Tumors of the kidney are much denser than benign lesions of the kidney, since the latter usually are cystic and filled with clear fluid. Moreover, the density of a kidney tumor is different from the adjacent normal kidney tissue, another means by which a malignancy can be detected.

The major role of CT scanning in urologic diagnosis is in determining the nature of masses within the kidney, but certainly patients with known prostatic cancer can be scanned with this modality. Indeed, it is often possible to determine the extent of the spread of a prostate cancer by means of CT scanning, particularly if the spread is extensive (Fig. 2–4). Sometimes, CT scans are obtained to try to see if there is evidence of lymph node involvement from the spread of the prostate cancer, but the high rate of false positives and false negatives when used for this purpose means that CT scans are not accurate or reliable enough for "staging" of cancer of the prostate (see below under "bone scanning"). For benign prostatic hyperplasia there are no indications for a CT scan; similarly, there are no indications for a CT scan in prostatic infection or inflammation.

Magnetic Resonance Imaging (MRI)

This very new imaging technique which relies heavily on computer assistance is somewhat similar to a CT scan in that cross-sectional images may be obtained. But this versatile and enormously expensive machine can also make images in the longitudinal, sagittal, and oblique planes. The method of obtaining the image is entirely different and there is one major improvement over CT scanning: the patient is not exposed to any radiation and there is therefore no known hazard to this study. Further, it is not necessary to introduce any contrast material into the bowel or the kidney in order to do the imaging (Fig. 2–5). The MRI image is seen on a screen and then transferred to photographic film. MRI offers much better diagnostic capabilities than CT scanning even though it is a

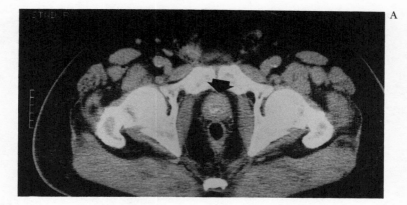

Figure 2–4   A. *A normal CT scan of the pelvis showing a normal prostate (arrow).*

B. A CT scan showing a greatly enlarged prostate with irregular margins due to a large and extensive prostate cancer (arrows). Both panels A and B are cross sections through the pelvis.

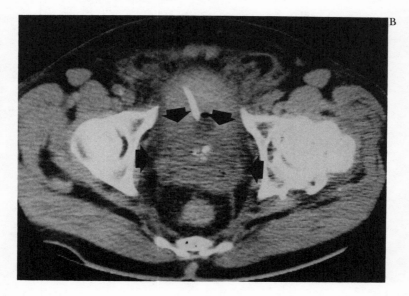

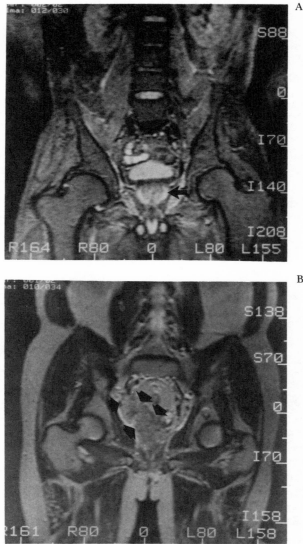

Figure 2–5 MAGNETIC RESONANCE IMAGING (MRI).

A. A normal prostate gland (arrow).

B. An extensive cancer of the prostate extending in an upward direction (arrows). Both panels A and B are longitudinal images through the pelvis.

new modality. Unquestionably, when MRI has been around as long as CT scanning has, it will probably replace most of the CT scanning devices now in use and will be the method of choice for imaging within the body. Its principle drawback is its prohibitive expense. New MRI machines generally cost well over two million dollars. MRI scanning of the prostate known to be malignant is sometimes done in the hope of determining whether the cancer has spread to the areas surrounding the prostate or to the lymph nodes in the pelvis. The scanning is best done with a coil in the rectum and it is perhaps somewhat more accurate than CT scanning for the same purpose; however, it cannot detect with accuracy whether or not the lymph nodes of the pelvis have cancer in them.

Bone Scanning and Bone X-rays

These are studies that are done when a diagnosis of prostatic carcinoma has been established or is strongly suspected. They are done for the purpose of "staging" the prostatic cancer. "Staging" is a medical term for the process of determining if a known cancer is still confined within the prostate and is therefore curable, or if it has spread outside the prostate gland and is probably not curable. One of the most common places to which prostate cancer spreads is to the bones, particularly those of the spine, the hips, the pelvis, and the long bones of the upper legs. When prostate cancer does spread to bone it damages and even destroys that bone to some degree. As soon as this damage or destruction has occurred, the body's natural healing process begins to lay down new bone in the damaged area.

If x-rays of the damaged bone are taken, the initial appearance is that of a "lytic" lesion, a medical term for the destructive process that makes the bone look as if it has virtually no substance and has a thinned-out appearance. As new bone is laid down by the body's natural healing process, it gives an x-ray appearance to the bone of being much denser than normal. This appearance is referred to as "blastic" (Fig. 2–6).

Obviously, there is a time lag between the time that

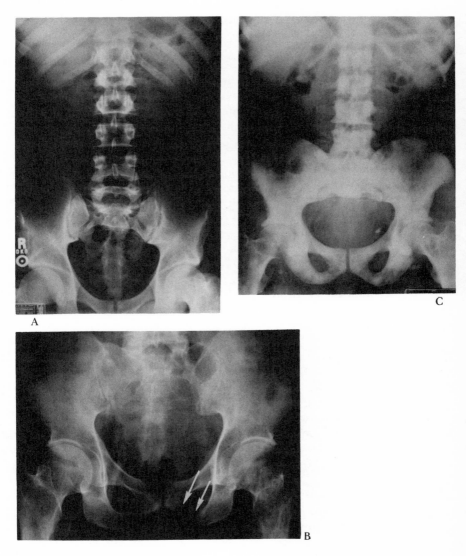

Figure 2–6 *A. Normal bone x-rays.*

B. Lytic lesion in the pubic bone (arrows) caused by virtually complete destruction of the bone from the spread of prostate cancer.

C. Blastic lesions diffusely seen through the spine and pelvis caused by the laying down of new bone secondary to extensive damage from the spread of prostate cancer.

destruction of the bone begins and the time when it first becomes visible on x-ray as either a lytic or a blastic lesion. However, between three and six months before anything at all is visible on x-ray, the changes that have occurred in bone from the spreading cancer can be visualized by means of bone scans which are much more sensitive at detecting early destruction and repair in bone than are x-rays. These scans are performed by injecting a radioisotope intravenously which then moves from the blood to the bone cells that are in a reparative phase. The amount of the radioisotope taken up by the bone is then actually counted by a device very similar to a Geiger counter which counts the amount of radioactivity (from the radioisotope) over the bone and displays each of these counts as a dot on a screen or a monitor. A bone that has had a heavy count of radioactivity over it can readily be visualized on the monitor and then on a piece of photographic paper to which it is transferred (Fig. 2–7). An increased number of counts of the radioisotope in one or more bony areas is considered to be strong presumptive evidence of the laying down of new bone in response to bone destruction. But it is not proof of the presence of cancer spread to bone. Any process that can destroy bone, such as an injury or even arthritis, will result in the initiation of the bone reparative mechanism, and this in turn will lead to an increased number of counts of radioactivity over those bony areas. In other words, a "positive" bone scan means only that bony destruction and the reparative process have occurred; it does *not* indicate what caused the bony destruction. However, if the isotope scans are compared with the bone x-rays and the areas of increased uptake are seen to have a perfectly normal appearance on x-ray (as opposed to an appearance of new or old trauma or arthritis), then the probability of metastatic cancer becomes the most likely diagnosis. Note that if the bone x-rays themselves show lytic or blastic lesions, there is no need to even do a bone scan.

Bone scans are not indicated in the management of patients with benign prostatic hyperplasia or with infection or inflammation of the prostate.

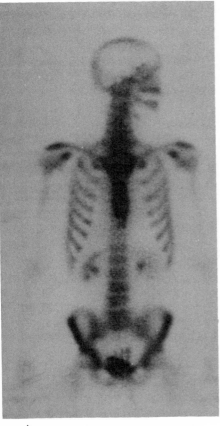
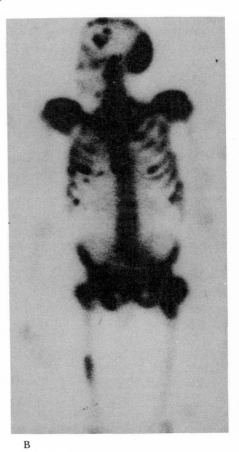

A   B

Figure 2–7 BONE SCANS

   A. A normal bone scan.

   B. A strongly positive bone scan with greatly increased uptake of radioisotope in many bones, particularly the skull, the shoulders, and the pelvis, all due to an extensive spread of cancer of the prostate to these bony areas.

Urodynamic Studies

The urinary bladder has two basic functions: urine storage and urine evacuation (voiding). Urodynamic studies are simply tests by which a physician is able to measure these functions as an objective means of evaluating the act of voiding and, more importantly, abnormalities of voiding. These urodynamic studies have many valuable functions in numerous urologic diseases, but the applicability of these studies to prostatic disease is fairly limited to the determination of the urinary flow rate. With benign prostatic hyperplasia (see Chapter 4) the natural history of the disease is such that the urinary stream becomes slower as the disease progresses. An objective measure of how obstructed the prostatic urethra is may be had by actually measuring the rate of urine flow through it. This can be done with a very fancy machine (Fig. 2–8) or simply with a stop watch and a measuring container which should nevertheless give a reasonable approximation of the true values. It must be recalled, however, that voiding is a function of both bladder contraction and the resistance to the flow of urine caused by the enlarged prostate. Therefore, an abnormally decreased urine flow rate does not prove that the problem is due to an enlarged and obstructing prostate. It may be due to poor bladder muscular condition, for example, and it is up to the physician to determine whether a decreased urinary flow rate is indicative of prostatic enlargement (which it usually is) or due to bladder muscle abnormalities (which is uncommon).

For an accurate urinary flow rate to be determined a voided volume of at least 150–200 ml is required. If the total volume voided is less than 100 ml the study is probably not valid. Nevertheless, with these caveats certain normal values for urinary flow rates have been well established, and when the urinary flow rate is under the generally accepted norm for a given patient's age group this may be regarded as an objective indication of bladder outlet obstruction. There are many men who simply cannot urinate if someone is watching them, even if that someone is a physician or a technician. For the accurate measurement of this voiding flow rate, however, it is not necessary for anyone to be present. Nevertheless, some men still

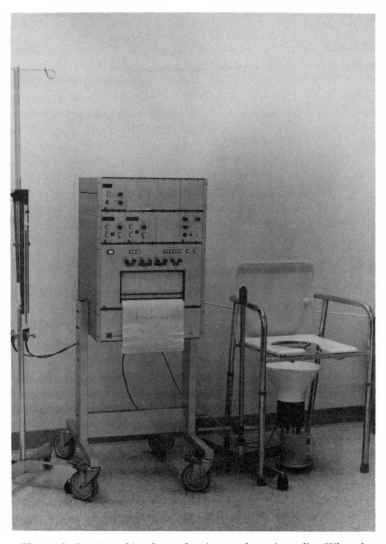

Figure 2–8   *A machine for performing urodynamic studies. When the study desired is a peak urine flow rate, the urine is voided into the commode-like apparatus on the right, the results are calculated with the machine on the left, and the results appear on the graph paper.*

have trouble initiating their stream knowing that they are being "tested" in some capacity or another. These men will undoubtedly have a considerable degree of hesitancy, a marked delay before they can initiate the urinary stream. However, once the stream is initiated, the nervousness is no longer a factor in the flow rate since the urinary stream, once begun, really just flows in an involuntary manner. So it is not at all difficult to get an accurate peak urine flow rate. I am sure there might be some individuals who simply cannot void in a test circumstance or whose voiding does not accurately reflect their maximum voiding ability. This would not greatly alter a final decision as to whether a patient does or does not have a mechanical obstruction to voiding (from his prostate) because there are many factors other than the flow rate that are taken into consideration in a diagnosis of BPH. Whether a patient has had too much or too little to drink is also immaterial as long as he is able to void at least 150–200 ml. If he is not, it may be helpful to give the patient several glasses of water to drink and then to repeat the study a couple of hours later. No specific preparation is usually necessary for this type of study.

Bladder Catheterization

Two distinct types of bladder catheterization are carried out and two distinct types of catheter are used (Fig. 2–9). One type is the "in-and-out" catheterization in which a catheter is put into the bladder for a very brief period of time in order to measure the amount of residual urine remaining immediately following voiding, an amount which is normally near

Figure 2–9 CATHETERS USED TO DRAIN THE BLADDER.
   A. A "straight" catheter that is used for "in-and-out" catheterization.
   B. A Foley catheter that is used when the catheter is to be left in the bladder for a period of time. The arrow points to the sidearm on the catheter through which a bag on the end of the catheter is inflated. The other portion of the catheter adjacent to the arrow is that part of the catheter through which urine drains, usually into a collecting bag.
   C. A Foley catheter with the bag on the end inflated (arrow). It is inflated after it has been placed inside the bladder, and the inflated bag catches on the inside of the bladder neck thereby preventing the catheter from falling out.

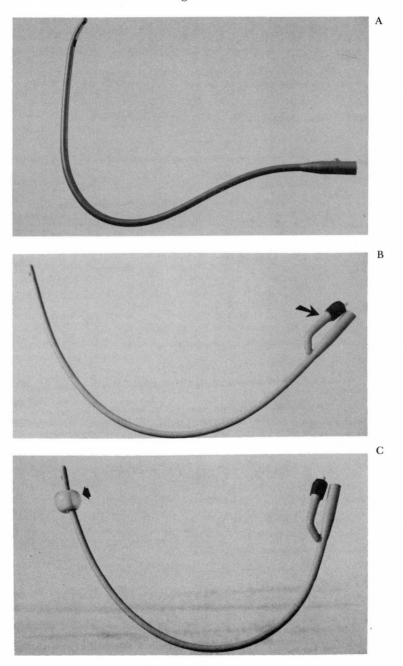

zero ml. However, when benign prostatic hyperplasia obstructs the bladder outlet, incomplete bladder emptying will usually occur eventually, and the larger the amount of residual urine left following voiding the more urgent the need for treatment and relief of the obstruction. "In-and-out" catheterization is also used to instill solutions into the bladder such as contrast medium for x-ray purposes or various medications for certain kinds of bladder disease. Yet another type of "in-and-out" catheterization is done intermittently several times per day for the individual who is unable to void at all because of a nerve deficiency such as may occur after an injury to the spinal cord.

The second broad category of catheterization is done with a special type of catheter which is then left indwelling in the bladder for long periods of time. This type of catheter, known as a Foley catheter, is able to stay inside the bladder because of a bag on its end that is inflated once the catheter is within the bladder thereby preventing the catheter from falling out. Long-term catheter drainage of this sort may be done for many different reasons, but for patients with prostatic enlargement it is done to facilitate continuous emptying of the bladder in individuals who are either totally unable to void because of the obstructing prostate tissue or who void so inefficiently that they leave behind large amounts of residual urine. As a general rule the indwelling catheter for these patients is left in place only until surgical correction of the obstructing prostate tissue can be carried out. Very rarely, continuous catheter drainage may go on indefinitely in a patient who refuses surgical treatment or whose general medical condition is so bad that he is not considered a suitable risk for surgery. The reason that the intermittent "in-and-out" type of catheterization is not done in these severely obstructed patients is because the obstructing prostate tissue in the prostatic urethra would make passage of the catheter difficult and traumatic if it were done several times a day for long periods of time.

As a urologist, I rarely think twice about catheterizing a patient when I feel it is in his best interest. Catheterization is a procedure that is so commonly and frequently done, by virtually all physicians, that I sometimes tend to overlook the extreme apprehension that can be brought on by the very *thought* of catheterization. I realize that when a catheterization is done it is neither painful nor harmful, but I am also a man and I can therefore understand the anxieties and concerns of my fellow men about an invasion of that most holy of holy parts of the male body. When a catheterization is necessary, whether it is in my office or in the hospital, I make a point of always explaining to my patient exactly what the procedure entails. Furthermore, I actually show him a catheter, exactly like the one that will be used, and tell him that the opening inside his penis is much, much larger than the catheter and therefore the procedure cannot possibly hurt him. I do, however, tell my patients that they may well find the procedure to be unpleasant. I have been catheterized myself and I tell this to my patients. I further tell them that the experience was far more unpleasant in contemplation than in the actual procedure which was not at all painful but which was mentally distressing simply because of the *thought* of what was being done to me. When I show the catheter to a patient, I make a point of having him feel it so that he can realize that it truly is made of soft rubber. I am convinced that this additional time spent with my patient prior to catheterization is time very well spent. When it is a Foley indwelling catheter that is being used, I will often actually show my patients exactly how the bag on the end of the catheter is inflated and then deflated and that neither of these acts will cause the patient any discomfort nor will removing the catheter when it is no longer needed. In actual fact, I do not think I can remember having a patient who has been properly prepared tell me that a catheterization, carefully done and using lots of lubricating jelly, has been painful or distressing or really anything more than a less-than-pleasant experience.

Cystoscopy

The diagnostic procedure that is most associated with the specialty of urology and with urologic disease is undoubtedly the cystoscopic examination of the bladder and the urethra. This examination is virtually the exclusive domain of urologists, and the precise and detailed knowledge obtained from it is but one example of how diagnostic techniques help to make urology the accurate and precise specialty that it is.

Cystoscopy involves the passage of a hollow instrument with a light and a lens on one end and a viewing lens on the other into the penile urethra and then into the bladder. Through the hollow instrument, urine that is in the bladder can run to the outside, thereby enabling the measurement of residual urine. After this procedure water is allowed to flow by gravity through the cystoscope *into* the bladder. This is necessary in order to inflate the bladder away from the lens end of the cystoscope. If you were to put your head inside a balloon you would have to inflate the balloon away from your eye in order to be able to see the interior of the balloon; for the same reason the bladder must be inflated away from the cystoscopic lens. Once the bladder is filled, it is possible to visualize with detail and accuracy the interior of the bladder. When visualizing the inside of the prostate gland and the inside of the urethra, it is not necessary to have the bladder inflated, because the inside of the prostate and the urethra are tubular in shape and more or less rigid whereas the bladder is a floppy structure that would simply collapse around the lens if it were not inflated.

Cystoscopes are generally rigid instruments, but recently flexible cystoscopes have been in use; the passage of these newer instruments into the bladder is similar to the passing of a catheter through the urethra and into the bladder (Fig. 2–10). With either instrument an anesthetic jelly is squirted into the urethra prior to passing the cystoscope. This sufficiently numbs the urethra so that patient discomfort is minimal and is actually much more mental than physical. I have always asked male patients after a cystoscopic exam with the rigid instrument how painful it was and invariably the reply has been that the thought of what was being done was far more unpleasant than the procedure itself.

By using a cystoscope the urologist is able to visualize the prostatic urethra and to diagnose inflammation of this area such as might be seen with nonspecific urethritis or even with chronic bacterial prostatitis if the infection / inflammation involved the prostatic urethra as well as the prostate (see Chapter 3). When a diagnosis of benign prostatic hyperplasia

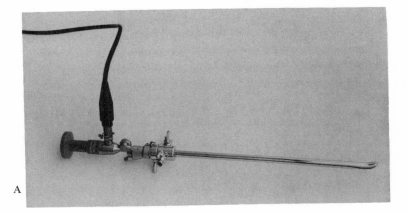

Figure 2-10   A. The standard cystoscope which is passed through the urethra and is used for visualizing the interior of the bladder and urethra. The black object attached to the cystoscope is the light cord.

B. The new and infrequently used flexible cystoscope which serves the same purpose as the standard cystoscope but may enable better visualization in certain hard-to-see parts of the bladder. Also it may be less uncomfortable for the patient because of its flexibility. Note that only the small, curved portion of the cystoscope (arrows) is introduced into the bladder. The light cord is seen leaving the cystoscope at the upper left.

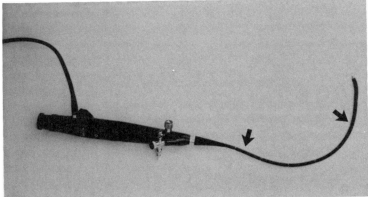

(BPH) is being considered (see Chapter 4), cystoscopy enables the urologist to evaluate and assess the degree of obstruction in the prostatic urethra, to estimate the size and weight of the obstructing prostatic tissue, and to make an accurate measurement of any residual urine which may be present in the bladder since this urine will come out through the cystoscope after it has entered the bladder. In patients with prostatic cancer, cystoscopy is used to locate sources of prostatic bleeding that tend to occur with this condition, and also to assess the degree of obstruction to the flow of urine caused by the cancerous growth that often, late in the course of the disease, obstructs the channel of the prostatic urethra.

It is perfectly natural for a man to be extremely apprehensive upon learning that he needs to be cystoscoped. This is partly because of anxiety over the unknown, but it is perhaps even more so because of the invasion of the sacred part of the male identity. A thoughtful physician is fully cognizant of this and will make every effort to make the procedure as non-threatening as possible and to make the patient as comfortable as possible. Occasionally, if the patient is not going to be driving a car right afterwards, an intravenous injection of a tranquilizing or a hypnotic agent prior to cystoscopy is helpful, but in my experience this is not usually necessary. I have very rarely used anything more than the requisite local anesthetic jelly instilled into the urethra along with a lot of reassurance and gentleness. The number of patients whom I have encountered over the years who have been unable to tolerate the procedure or who have said afterwards that they wished that they had been put to sleep or given an injection have been few and far between and have numbered well under one percent of all patients.

Prostatic Aspirations and Prostatic Biopsies

These diagnostic tests are used whenever carcinoma of the prostate is suspected, a suspicion that may be triggered by several things. Most often, it is aroused when a digital rectal examination of the prostate gland discloses an area that is noticeably firmer than the surrounding gland. Sometimes, this may be an asymmetric enlargement of the prostate gland, which raises the question in the examining physician's mind of a possible malignancy (Fig. 2–11A). A biopsy should also be considered when there is an elevation of the PSA blood test. Suspicion should also be aroused when a patient gives a history of bladder outlet obstruction that sounds suggestive of benign prostatic hyperplasia but in which the duration of symptoms is very brief, perhaps three to six months or less. Inasmuch as the typical patient with BPH will have had his symptoms for several years prior to seeing the physician, a relatively sudden onset of symptoms of bladder outlet obstruction should alert the physician to the possibility of a rapidly growing carcinoma of the prostate that is encroaching upon and obstructing the prostatic urethra, *regardless* of the feel of the prostate on digital rectal examination. Finally, suspicion should be aroused by a patient who visits his physician because of severe pain in a bone and whose x-rays and / or bone scans suggest the possibility of bone destruction from some sort of cancer. In the search for the origin of cancer that has spread to bone the prostate must always be high on the suspect list. The alert physician may recommend prostatic biopsies or aspirations even if the prostate has a relatively normal feel to it.

Needle Aspiration of the Prostate Gland

This relatively painless procedure for determining the presence or absence of prostatic cancer was originally used more than fifty years ago but never achieved any degree of popularity because of the difficulty in interpreting the specimen material that was obtained from the prostate. The material consists of individual cells or clumps of cells that are literally aspirated or sucked out of the prostate gland through a very thin or "skinny" needle, a very different method from the classic prostate biopsy in which a plug or core of tissue is removed. In the very recent past, however, due to the increasing excellence of the pathologists who read and interpret the specimens, the skinny-needle prostate aspiration technique has become a highly accurate means of determining the presence or absence of prostate cancer. As recently as five years ago the technique was sophisticated enough to say with certainty if a

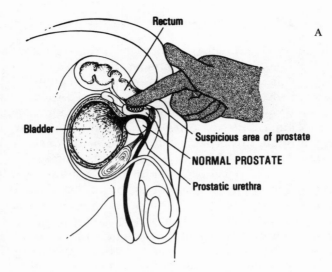

Figure 2–11   *A. Shows the examining finger in the rectum feeling a hard or suspicious area of the prostate gland.*

B. The same view, but now there is a tru-cut biopsy needle in the hand of the examining physician, positioned right over the suspicious hard part of the prostate gland preparatory to taking a biopsy of the area. The same positioning is used with the aspiration technique when the skinny needle is used instead of the tru-cut needle.

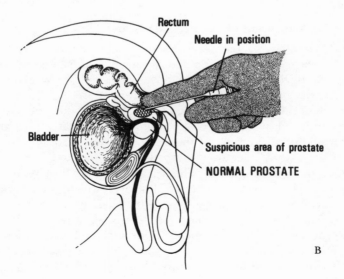

highly malignant prostatic cancer existed but it was not sufficiently developed to differentiate between a low-grade prostate cancer and benign prostatic hyperplasia. Very recently,
however, the technique and particularly the means of interpretation have been refined to the point that a skilled cyto-
pathologist (a physician trained as a pathologist with special
training in the appearance of cells) can now say with certainty
whether the removed aspirate is benign, of low-grade malignancy, or of high-grade malignancy.

The skinny-needle aspiration biopsy is performed with the
patient on his knees on an examining table with his head resting on a pillow. A prophylactic dose of an oral antibiotic is
given to minimize the chances of infection since rectal bacteria may be introduced into the prostate. The physician's index
finger is inserted in the rectum and placed over the area of
the prostate that is suspicious for the possibility of malignancy. A long, thin, hollow needle is concealed just inside the
crook of the physician's index finger until the finger has definitely identified the area of the prostate that is suspicious for
malignancy. The syringe and skinny needle are then advanced
as the index finger is slightly elevated to permit this and the
needle is directed right through the rectum and into the part
of the prostate that is to be aspirated. This is done while the
tip of the index finger is in very close proximity to the suspicious area so that the physician can be certain that the needle
has been directed properly (Fig. 2–11B). Once the needle is
in the area to be aspirated a negative suction is developed
within the syringe, a very small amount of material is sucked
up into the needle, and is placed onto a slide once the needle
has been removed from the patient. This material is then
examined by an experienced cell pathologist and the results
are rapidly available to the examining physician.

In recent years I have performed many of these skinny-
needle prostatic aspirations and resident urologists working
with me have performed even more. None of us have ever
heard a patient say that the procedure is any more painful or
uncomfortable than a needle injected into the arm or but-
tocks when medication is given. No anesthesia is necessary
and that, of course, is one of the enormous advantages of this
type of biopsy. The big advantage of the "skinny" needle—

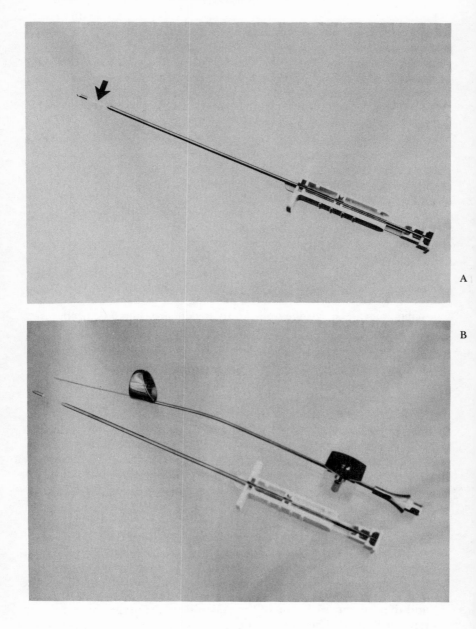

A

B

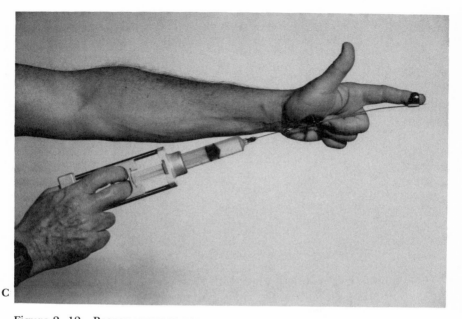

Figure 2–12 Biopsy needles used for the prostate gland.

A. *The tru-cut needle which is most commonly used for the pro-state biopsies. A core or plug of prostate tissue is obtained within the hollow portion (arrow) of this needle.*

B. *The tru-cut needle (below) and the skinny needle which is used for aspirating cells from the prostate gland for diagnostic purposes.*

C. *The actual position of the skinny needle during a prostatic aspiration. The physician's finger would be in the rectum pressing on the suspicious area of prostate gland into which the skinny needle would then be directed. The physician's other hand exerts significant negative pressure with the pistol-grip type of aspiration device enabling prostatic cells to be sucked out of the prostate and into the syringe.*

lack of pain—has now largely been obliterated by the spring-loaded biopsy "guns" which are so rapid that they are virtually painless; they also provide much more tissue—and therefore the potential for greater diagnostic accuracy—for the pathologist to examine.

Prostatic Biopsy

The traditional method for many years of establishing the diagnosis of prostatic cancer has been the "tru-cut" biopsy method: the use of a large, hollow needle by means of which a core or plug of prostate tissue perhaps a millimeter in diameter and a couple of centimeters long is removed. (Fig. 2–12) Microscopic examination of the removed prostatic tissue requires the services of a competent pathologist, but it does not require the additional skills of a specially trained cell pathologist. Since these very highly trained cell pathologists are not always available in smaller hospitals, the more standard technique of obtaining a core or plug of tissue for examination is still used and is still an excellent technique. It is also indicated in those situations where the aspiration technique gives equivocal or indeterminate results.

The core or plug biopsy technique using the large needle is basically similar to that of the aspiration technique as far as the method by which the needle is introduced into the prostate gland through the rectum. Using the large "core" biopsy needle—with or without the spring-loaded biopsy "gun"—a much larger hole is placed into the rectum and the prostate, thereby increasing the risk of infection. For this reason antibiotics and cleansing enemas / laxatives are given the night before and / or one to two days after the biopsy.

Because of this complication with infections when the approach through the rectum is used, some urologists prefer to direct the large biopsy needle through the perineum (the area between the anus and the scrotum) and into the prostate gland, attempting to direct the needle to the suspicious part of the prostate by keeping an index finger in the rectum and feeling the prostate gland as the needle is pushed through the tissues of the perineum. I feel that such biopsies should only be considered reliable if they are positive for cancer and that a negative biopsy must invariably lead to the strong possibility that the suspicious area was not the area actually biopsied because of the difficulty in doing biopsies accurately through the tissues of the perineum.

As noted above under the section on ultrasound, the most commonly used method for doing biopsies of the prostate has been the use of ultrasound combined with the spring-loaded biopsy "gun." With this method, the ultrasound probe in the rectum (Fig. 2–13) is used (by the physician watching a screen) to guide the biopsy needle into the suspicious area of the

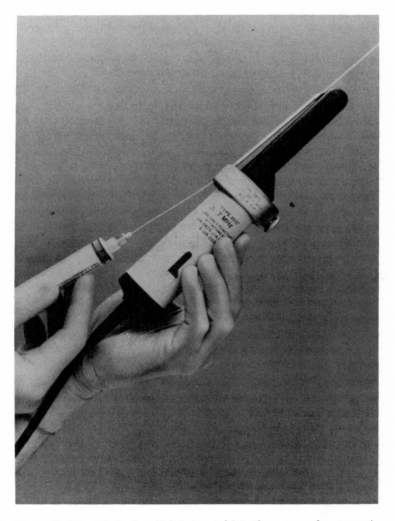

Figure 2–13   *The probe which is inserted into the rectum when prostatic "Ultrasound" is done. It is this probe which sends out the high-frequency sound waves and which then "listens" for the echo response (see the section on ultrasound in this chapter). The needle, which is seen alongside the probe, is one kind that is used for the prostate biopsy. (Photograph through the courtesy of Brüel and Kjaer Instruments, Inc., Marlborough, Massachusetts.)*

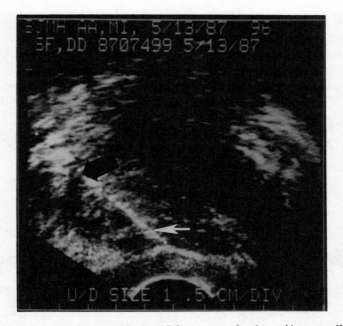

Figure 2–14 *Ultrasound image of the prostate showing a biopsy needle within the prostate gland. This biopsy needle appears as a straight-line, white area in the lower left portion of the photograph (white arrow). The tip of the needle is obtaining a biopsy from within a less dense area of the prostate (black arrow) that may possibly have cancer within it. (Photograph through the courtesy of Brüel and Kjaer Instruments, Inc., Marlborough, Massachusetts.)*

prostate. The biopsy needle is directed through the rectum and can be seen on the screen as it is advanced right up to the suspicious area of the prostate (Figs. 2–14 and 2–15). The biopsy "gun" is then fired and the action of the biopsy needle is so rapid that it is actually painless.

Prostate biopsy, with any technique, is not indicated for the patient considered to have benign prostatic hyperplasia or inflammation / infection in the prostate gland.

Following prostate biopsy it is not rare to have some blood appear in the urine or in the semen during ejaculation. This simply means that the biopsy needle entered the inside of the

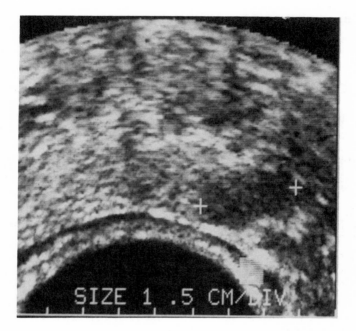

Figure 2–15 *An ultrasound image of the prostate gland. Note the area at the bottom right which is between the two small cross-marks. This area is less dense than the surrounding portion of the prostate gland. It is an area such as this which is felt to possibly have cancer within it and which would therefore be biopsied. (Photograph through the courtesy of Brüel and Kjaer Instruments, Inc., Marlborough, Massachusetts.)*

prostatic urethra during the course of the biopsy; it is not a cause for worry or alarm. The bleeding will usually stop after a day or two, but if it is heavy or lasts beyond a couple of days you should tell your urologist. Blood in the semen may last for a number of ejaculations because each time you ejaculate you cause a violent spasm of the muslces inside your urethra (what propels the semen to the outside). This spasm can cause the bleeding to recur before the area is finally healed. If you see blood in the ejaculate it is probably best to avoid ejaculation for several days in order to let the affected parts heal.

Interpretation of Prostate Biopsy

Once the biopsy has been done the obvious question to be answered is a yes or no as to whether or not cancer is present. Beyond this, and of great importance as far as being one of several factors in predicting success of therapy, is the actual microscopic appearance of the cancer. Is it high grade (very malignant) or relatively low grade (less malignant)? One very common method that pathologists use to determine and report this is the Gleason scale. Using this method, the pathologist grades the cancer as seen on a 1–5 scale of increasing malignancy and grades separately both the cancer pattern most commonly seen and the cancer pattern that appears to be secondary (often these will both be the same). These two numbers are then noted and added together to give the Gleason score, i.e. 3/3 or 6. Total scores of 2, 3, and 4 are considered low grade (less malignant) cancers; scores of 5, 6, and 7 are of intermediate malignancy, and scores of 8, 9, and 10 are highly malignant. Some pathologists choose to report biopsies simply as Grade I (Gleason 2,3,4), Grade II (Gleason 5,6,7) or Grade III (Gleason 8,9,10). Still other pathologists prefer to use a 1–4 scale with 1 being the least malignant and 4 the most malignant.

A special situation in which detection of prostate cancer can be somewhat more difficult is that in which a man has had surgery on his intestinal tract and is left with no rectum at all. In this case it is obviously impossible to do a digital rectal exam in order to feel the prostate gland and so the early suspicion and detection of prostate cancer must be based solely on the PSA blood level. If this level is such that your doctor is concerned about the possibility of prostate cancer, he can order a CT scan of your lower abdomen and the radiologist is able to guide a series of needle biopsies of your prostate using the CT image for control of the biopsy needle. This is a perfectly satisfactory method of performing a prostate biopsy in these circumstances.

3

Infection and Inflammation in the Prostate Gland (and the Prostatic Urethra)

RLM, a 31-year-old architect, came to my office recently in an obvious state of extreme mental anguish. He had called my office earlier that day and had been told that I had no available time in my schedule until later in the week. He pleaded with my office secretary to allow him to come in that very day, saying that it was extremely urgent and all but telling her that it was a matter of "life or death."

When I saw him later that same afternoon, he was clearly distraught, but yet he was obviously in no particular pain or discomfort and appeared to be in excellent health.

"Doctor," he started out, "Something is very wrong and I am frankly scared stiff of what might happen because of it."

It didn't take me very long to find out that this man had two symptoms and a lot of resulting worries. First, he had noticed a dime-sized brownish stain inside his shorts when he undressed before retiring the previous night. Second, he had noticed that the opening on the end of his penis seemed to be glued into a shut position when he woke up that morning. When he pulled apart the two sides of this opening he noticed a tiny drop of very clear fluid just inside. He had no pain, no discomfort on voiding, did not feel sick, and maintained his usual state of good health. Regardless, he became quite frantic and remained so until his visit to my office. His fears centered around the perceived complications that could result from these two minor symptoms. He was specifically worried that he might develop cancer of the prostate or benign prostatic hyperplasia, but his most severe concern was that his present problem could lead to impotence. This patient was unmarried and had a moderately active sex life compatible with the great time demands of his profession. He had never had anything like this before, he said.

This man's symptoms and problems were common. Indeed, it has been my experience that there is probably no other single group of genitourinary tract symptoms that brings so many patients to the urologist, and probably to the primary care physician as well, as those of infection and inflammation in the prostate gland and in the prostatic urethra. With some exceptions, these different disorders tend to produce rather similar symptoms—with many variations—and it is not an exaggeration to state that there is no other group of disorders, real or imagined, to which young and middle-aged males fall prey that causes more worry, anxiety, and concern than these ailments. In this particular example, my patient had a very mild infection in his prostatic urethra; his anguish well reflects the fact that the concerns and the anxiety that develop in these patients are enormously out of proportion to the severity of the illness and equally out of proportion to the severity of the symptoms. I love to make the analogy between a minimal discharge from the urethra, or even an itch or some discomfort in the urethra on the one hand, and a runny nose or an itchy or sore throat on the other. The latter group of symptoms could be present for months or even years without resulting in a patient visiting his physician, but the former group of symptoms need only be present for a few hours before a very worried and frightened patient comes running to a physician.

Because of the anatomic relationship of the prostatic urethra to the prostate gland (see Chapter 1), disease in either can produce symptoms that are similar, that overlap, and that at times can be virtually identical. Although the symptoms of the patient just cited were caused by a mild infection in the prostatic urethra, known as a nonspecific urethritis (NSU), his symptoms would not have been very different if he instead had suffered from a mild inflammation of the prostate gland caused by bacterial infection (chronic bacterial prostatitis), or a mild inflammation of the prostate gland *not* caused by bacteria (chronic nonbacterial prostatitis). This latter condition is also known as prostatostasis because it is felt that this condition is caused by a stasis, an inadequate emptying of fluids normally manufactured in the prostate gland.

When infection and inflammation in the prostatic urethra are present, any or all of the following symptoms may also be present: 1) a very minimal, watery discharge at the opening on the end of the penis seen mainly on arising in the morning. Sometimes, this minimal discharge causes the opening to be "glued" shut; 2) a brownish or yellowish stain about the size of a dime or a quarter noted inside the shorts at the end of the day; 3) an itching feeling inside the penis; 4) a feeling of discomfort within the penis on voiding; and 5) a feeling of discomfort or itching deep inside the penis in what would actually be the prostatic urethra. This infection and inflammation, nonspecific urethritis, is due to *any* kind of infection or inflammation of the prostatic and adjacent portions of the urethra *except* that caused by the gonococcus organism (gonorrhea). Gonorrhea affects the anterior portion of the urethra (that part of the urethra enclosed within the penis), while nonspecific urethritis typically affects the posterior portion of the urethra, predominantly made up of that portion of the urethra that is within the prostate gland (see Fig. 1–3). Infection and inflammation within the prostatic urethra most often are caused by a virus-like organism, chlamydia; but there are other organisms, virtually all of which are transmitted through oral, vaginal, or anal intercourse, that can produce the symptoms of nonspecific urethritis.

The symptoms of bacterial infection and nonbacterial inflammation of the prostate may occasionally include any or all of those just noted. In addition, there are usually symptoms of pain or discomfort in the perineum (the area between the scrotum and the anus), in the rectum, or in the area just above the pubic hair line (the suprapubic area). Prostatodynia is another condition that is similar in symptomatology, but it is a condition in which the prostate itself is probably normal. Patients usually attribute their pain or discomfort in the perineum and / or rectum to prostatitis because some physician or other in the past erroneously told them that they had prostatitis. Because of the great similarity of symptoms between four very different problems (nonspecific urethritis, chronic bacterial prostatitis, chronic nonbacterial prostatitis, and prostatodynia), it is absolutely imperative that a physician follow very specific diagnostic guidelines so as to be certain of the correctness of a diagnosis before it is rendered. Diseases of the genital structures are of overwhelming importance to most men, and an erroneous or misleading diagnosis can lead to needless anguish and anxiety and sometimes even to medical complications.

If you are confused about the difference between infection and inflammation, you are in good company, for many physicians are similarly confused. Though the symptoms of each and the effect of each on a given part of the body can be identical, "infection" means that bacteria or some other microorganism is the cause of the disease, while "inflammation" means that the disease is caused by factors *other than* bacteria or some other microorganism. Infection will rarely occur without inflammation, but inflammation will often occur without infection. Obvious causes of inflammation *without* infection are heat (sunburn), x-rays (radiation), and chemicals (a lye burn). Chronic bacterial prostatitis results from bacterial infection in the prostate, while chronic nonbacterial inflammation of the prostate has never been associated with bacteria and is presumably associated with engorgement or inadequate emptying of the prostate gland (prostatostasis).

Chronic bacterial infection in the prostate (chronic bacterial prostatitis) probably results from residual infection following inadequate or incomplete treatment of an episode of acute bacterial infection in the prostate (see acute bacterial prostatitis, below). In my experience, patients with this problem are often able to recall an earlier bout of acute bacterial prostatitis. Undoubtedly, chronic bacterial infection in the prostate can also be caused by bacteria entering the prostate gland from areas of infection within the prostatic urethra. It is also theoretically possible for bacteria to reach the prostate gland by a spread through the bloodstream from a focus of bacterial infection in a distant part of the body such as the skin, the ears, the teeth, or the tonsils. This type of blood-borne seeding of the prostate gland is very uncommon and some urologists question its occurrence at all.

Chronic nonbacterial inflammation of the prostate produces symptoms very much like those of chronic bacterial prostatic infection, but this inflammation is a condition in which it has never been possible, with any degree of consistency, to demonstrate any bacteria or other kind of microorganism within the prostate. I feel that the symptoms of this nonbacterial condition probably result from an engorgement of the fluid-producing glands within the prostate itself; this in turn results from irregular or infrequent emptying of the prostate gland. The prostate gland is emptied during orgasm and ejaculation by spasmodic contractions of the muscles around it, in much the same way that a sponge is emptied when it is squeezed. If a man is used to ejaculating on a fairly regular basis of one, two, three, or more times weekly and then, for whatever reason, his frequency of orgasm and ejaculation decreases sharply, it is likely that his prostate gland will become overly full of fluid. Although it is certainly a possibility that at some future time the condition that we now know as chronic nonbacterial prostatitis (prostatostasis) may be linked to bacterial organisms within the prostate gland that have thus far avoided isolation and identification, it is certainly true that as of this writing no such organisms have been discovered by intense research efforts. Therefore, the very plausible concept of nonbacterial prostatitis being caused by a prostatic engorgement is the one that is currently accepted.

Prostatodynia is a condition in which pain is perceived in the perineum or rectum, conceivably originating in the prostate, but much more likely coming from the muscles of the floor of the pelvis, from an inflammation in one or more of the pelvic bones, or from a disease process in the rectum.

Individuals having the condition of prostatodynia have no demonstrable abnormalities within the prostate gland.

Even though each of the foregoing conditions produces similar and sometimes even overlapping symptoms, they are each distinct entities that must be identified and correctly diagnosed because the treatment is very different for each of these conditions. A serious injury to a patient's mental or physical well-being may well result if a physician does not correctly diagnose the problem and treat it accordingly.

Diagnostic Studies Used to Differentiate between Chronic Bacterial and Nonbacterial Prostatitis and Nonspecific Urethritis

When a patient has some or all of the symptoms just noted, the two likeliest diagnoses are chronic nonbacterial prostatitis and nonspecific urethritis. The former would be the first-choice diagnosis in the relative absence of any sort of discharge from the urethra; the latter would be the best bet in the presence of a minimal and watery urethral discharge. Chronic bacterial prostatitis and prostatodynia are very long shots since these conditions are much less common. Nevertheless, making the correct diagnosis is not a matter of playing the odds, but is very precise and accurate if the examining physician will only take the time and trouble to follow the necessary steps in order to arrive at the correct diagnosis. This is something, in my experience, that is rarely done.

Physical examination is of little help in distinguishing between chronic bacterial prostatitis, chronic nonbacterial prostatitis (prostatostasis), and prostatodynia. I become distressed when a physician (and this often includes even urologists) performs a digital rectal examination on a patient with some or many of the symptoms already noted and then makes a diagnosis of chronic bacterial "infection in the prostate" based upon the finding of an "enlarged," a "soft," or a "boggy" prostate gland. This is absolutely fallacious reasoning because the softness or bogginess of the prostate gland in most men depends entirely upon the recent frequency of orgasm and ejaculations. The prostate gland is normally sponge-like and full of numerous small glands that produce about 80 percent of the fluid present in the ejaculate. If an individual who customarily ejaculates several times per week has a sudden change of habit so that he ejaculates once weekly or even less frequently, it should be obvious that the prostate will feel somewhat larger and softer than normally because it is engorged with prostatic fluid. In other words, the finding on digital rectal examination of a somewhat enlarged or boggy prostate gland should suggest only that the prostate gland is engorged because of infrequent ejaculations, and it should absolutely not cause the examining physician to proclaim that the patient has prostatitis unless it is clearly defined as nonbacterial prostatitis. All such patients with any, some, or all of the symptoms under discussion should properly have a bacterial localization test which will enable the physician, with certainty, to determine whether or not there is an infection in the prostate gland, in the urethra, or, as is much more frequently the case, nowhere at all (Fig. 3–1).

The patient is asked to begin urinating into a glass marked #1; then, without interrupting his stream, he is asked to void a couple of ounces into the toilet and then a couple of ounces of urine into a glass marked #2; then, again without interrupting his steam, he can void into the toilet while still consciously retaining some urine in his bladder. The physician then vigorously massages ("strips") the prostate gland to force prostatic fluid (secretions) out of the prostate gland and into the prostatic urethra. This vigorous massage or stripping of the prostate gland is not a painful procedure but is not a pleasant one, either. The discomfort that it may cause varies greatly from patient to patient because the sensitivity of the prostate gland to touch will also vary greatly from patient to patient. The prostatic stripping is done with a patient bent sharply at the waist and leaning over a table so that the physician can easily insert his finger into the rectum. The physician then places his finger on one side of the prostate gland and rolls his finger inward pressing very firmly downward as he rolls his finger from the outside margin of the prostate

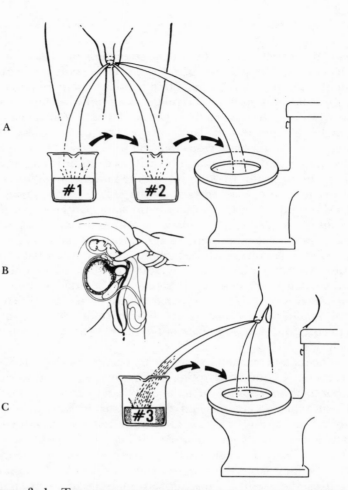

Figure 3–1 TECHNIQUE FOR LOCALIZING THE SOURCE OF INFECTION
TO THE URETHRA OR TO THE PROSTATE.

A. *This illustrates a patient starting his urinary stream in glass #1,
continuing it in glass #2 (midstream urine), and finishing it in the toilet,
leaving some urine remaining in the bladder.*

B. *This shows the prostate being massaged or "stripped" by the physician. Note a drop or two of prostatic secretions coming out of the penile
urethra.*

C. *This shows glass #3 which represents the first ounce or two of voiding immediately following the prostatic massage. Glass #3 will contain
most of the secretions from the prostate gland. The patient then finishes this
voiding into the toilet.*

gland towards the middle of the prostate gland. He then moves his finger to the outside margin on the other side of the prostate gland and does the same thing. Each of the two sides of the prostate gland is thus massaged or stripped about ten or twelve times. This downward pressure by the physician's finger serves to squeeze the fluid that is normally within the prostate gland out through the various prostatic ducts and into the middle of the prostatic urethra where it pools.

While the prostatic massaging or stripping is being done, the patient will often feel that fluid is trying to come out of his penis; this sensation is caused by the prostatic fluid (secretions) pooling in the prostatic urethra. The patient should keep his urethra squeezed shut with his hand. At the end of the prostate "massage" these expressed prostatic secretions may travel down the urethra and through the opening at the end of the penis where they may be collected for culture. Usually, however, the prostatic secretions remain pooled in the prostatic urethra, and the patient is again asked to begin to urinate after the stripping is complete, to void an ounce or two into a glass marked #3. He is then allowed to finish emptying his bladder into the toilet. Glass #3, or the actual prostatic secretions if they come out of the opening on the end of the penis, represent secretions from the interior of the prostate gland. A definitive diagnosis of chronic bacterial prostatitis can then be made if there is at least a tenfold increase in the bacterial colony count obtained from the urine in glass #3 as compared with glass #1, while the culture of urine in glass #2 (the midstream specimen) must be sterile. The bacterial counts for which one is searching in this localization test are in the neighborhood of a few hundred to a few thousand colonies of bacteria per milliliter of urine. A positive test for chronic bacterial prostatitis would show something like 3,000 colonies of bacteria in glass #3 and 300 colonies of bacteria in glass #1. If the bacterial colony count is the same in glass #1 as in glass #3, or if the colony count is greater in glass #1 than in glass #3, then the likely diagnosis is a nonspecific urethritis. Most frequently, in my experience, there are no bacteria found in any of the three specimens, thereby eliminating the diagnosis of chronic bacterial prostatitis or nonspecific urethritis, and leaving as the most probable diagnosis that of chronic nonbacterial prostatitis.

To sum up, I believe that it is absolutely erroneous for a physician to diagnosis chronic bacterial prostatitis unless either: 1) the bacterial colony count in glass #3 exceeds the colony count in glass #1 by a factor of at least ten; or 2) the expressed prostatic secretions yield a positive bacterial culture with a colony count tenfold higher than the colony count in glass #1.

Should the bladder urine (glass #2) be infected, the entire bacterial localization test must be repeated after the urine has been sterilized with an antibiotic. I personally like to use nitrofurantoin (Macrodantin) for this purpose because this particular antibiotic is excellent for clearing up infections in the urine. It does not, however, penetrate into the prostate gland and therefore cannot interfere with the accurate determination of whether there are bacteria within the prostate gland. It is important to do this sterilization of the bladder urine because the presence of bacteria in the bladder urine can distort the results of the bacterial localization test. In fact, however, if the midstream urine (glass #2) is positive for infection (in the case of bladder urine a positive colony count would have more than 50,000 or 100,000 colonies of bacteria per milliliter of urine), the diagnosis of chronic bacterial prostatitis is indeed very likely. Conversely, if a patient has never had any documented infections of his bladder urine during any of the periods that he has had his symptoms of prostatic disease, the odds are overwhelming that he does not have and never has had chronic bacterial infection in his prostate gland.

At the time of the prostatic massage, if any of the prostatic fluid does travel down the urethra and outside of the penis, it is obtained for culture and (of great importance) is placed on a slide for microscopic examination. When this is done, and when a true chronic bacterial prostatitis exists, the prostatic fluid will usually have more than 20 white blood cells (pus cells) per high power microscopic field, and these will usually appear in clumps. There may also be an increase seen in the amount of fat present, and this fat is seen contained within large cells called macrophages. Unfortunately, these findings are also found when a diagnosis of nonbacterial prostatitis (prostatostasis) exists. The only sure way of differentiating between these two conditions is by culturing the expressed prostatic secretions or the urine that is produced immediately following prostatic massage. Bacteria will be found in the secretions of patients having bacterial prostatitis, and no bacteria will be found in the secretions of patients having non-bacterial prostatitis. In the patient with prostatodynia, and also in any normal and asymptomatic patient, there will usually be fewer than 10 white blood cells per high power field, and they will not appear in clumps.

Treatment of Prostatic Infection and Inflammation

The treatment of each of these conditions is quite different and distinct from the treatment of the other conditions; therefore it is imperative that the correct diagnosis be made. Nonspecific urethritis is usually treated with antibiotics such as tetracycline, or with one of the synthetic tetracyclines such as Doxycycline or Minocycline. Chronic bacterial prostatitis is usually treated with a combination of sulfa and trimethoprim (Bactrim or Septra), with carbenicillin (Geocillin), or with one of the fluoroquinolones (a new group of antibiotics) such as Noroxin or Cipro, depending upon the sensitivity to antibiotics of the specific bacterial organism found in the cultures. Nonbacterial prostatitis (prostatostasis) is best treated without antibiotics by encouraging a frequent emptying of the prostate gland via increased frequency of masturbation, intercourse, or both. Inasmuch as the reason for the patient's symptoms is a prostate that has become fluid-laden because of irregular and / or infrequent ejaculations, the therapy of this condition is sensible and certainly not unpleasant. Clearly, prostatic massage can produce similar results as far as emptying the prostate gland of its excess secretions, but I generally condemn this when it is done more than a total of three or four times. I refer to it then as chronic "remunerative" prostatitis because I feel that it serves no particular purpose other than to separate the patient from his money. It is really quite unnecessary unless the patient is physically or emotionally unable to masturbate or have intercourse. Prostatodynia, which is not truly a disease of the prostate gland itself, is usually treated symptomatically with muscle relaxants to relieve muscle spasms of the musculature of the floor of the pelvis along with such remedies as hot sitz baths and even occasionally tranquilizers. I have also on occasion used nonsteroidal anti-inflammatory agents such as Motrin for prostatodynia; this is based upon studies showing that some of these patients apparently have an inflammation in the pubic bone that seems to respond to the anti-inflammatory type of management.

Unfortunately, because of the specific parts of the body that are affected, infection and inflammation of the prostate and urethra cannot be managed in nearly as straightforward a manner as can infection or inflammation elsewhere in the body. The physician must be extremely cautious and circumspect in diagnosing and treating patients who might have one of these conditions. I have said before that there is but one giant synapse between a man's genitals and his brain, and the thought that anything could be wrong with the prostate gland (considered to be a genital structure) is anathema to many men and brings stark fear and severe apprehension to most others. In my experience, once a physician has told a patient that he has prostatitis, it is inevitable that the same physician will put the patient on some antibiotic. In the patient's own mind the diagnosis of prostatitis combined with the antibiotics sends him a very strong signal that he has a bacterial infection in his prostate gland. To be sure, the physician undoubtedly really believes that a bacterial infection *does* exist despite the fact that very few physicians take the time or the trouble to do the three-glass culture method outlined; they just assume the presence of a bacterial infection.

The vast majority of patients so treated will not show any improvement in their symptoms because there is no infection and no bacteria present. The net effect of the unsuccessful antibiotic therapy is to worry the patient and exacerbate his concern that he is not getting any better. Most men who did not have a bacterial infection but are managed in this manner will continue to have their symptoms for a long period of time, and will usually have a recurring problem of "prostatitis" for many years after the original diagnosis was made. Whenever any symptoms in the general anatomic area of the prostate gland occur the patient's level of anxiety and concern will skyrocket and he will be convinced that his "infection in the prostate" has returned. Sadly, his physician will usually concur and the cycle of inappropriate antibiotic therapy compounded by genuine anxiety begins again. Moreover, by diagnosing "prostatitis" and treating for an infection when none exists, the physician is putting the patient's health at risk because of the antibiotics themselves. When these drugs are prescribed for a prostatic "infection," patients will usually remain on them for many months while anticipating the symptomatic relief that will never come. It is not at all rare for a patient to develop allergic manifestations to the antibiotics, some of which can be life-threatening. Such severe reactions represent an unfortunate situation if the antibiotics were truly needed, but it is an absolutely tragic situation when the antibiotics should never have been prescribed in the first place!

I am often reminded of a near tragedy that occurred when one of my faculty colleagues at my previous university turned up in the urology department one day complaining of a vague discomfort when he voided and a vague ache in his perineum. This gentleman, a 45-year-old full professor of medicine, was absolutely convinced that he had prostatitis, and he was equally convinced that antibiotics were required for his problem. One of my colleagues in the urology department saw him, examined him, did a bacterial localization test, and told him that he definitely did not have any evidence of bacterial infection in the prostate and antibiotics were not indicated. Unfortunately, this rather headstrong professor of medicine, who had just enough knowledge of urologic problems to be dangerous to himself, went to another urologist practicing in the community and gave the same story. He was promptly put on a course of an antibiotic which contained sulfa and within a week was hospitalized for the next six weeks with a generalized sloughing of the lining of his mouth and his intestinal tract. This is a very well-known and dreaded complication of sulfa therapy, but happily the patient recovered eventually. However, his prostatic symptoms continued and he next came to see me. My examination fully confirmed the impression of my colleague who had felt there was no evidence for antibiotic therapy because there was no evidence of bacterial infection. The professor of medicine and I spent the next half hour discussing his situation, while I probed into other possible symptoms he might have. His ongoing extramarital affair soon came to light. I will never be able to prove that his feelings of guilt because of this affair caused the symptoms which he associated with prostatic infection, but his symptoms did disappear within a couple of weeks after I pointed out this possibility to him.

I cannot say that the case example just cited is typical or even common, but I am quite certain that the psyche is able to produce an infinite variety of bodily symptoms, and I am equally certain that the male perception of the prostate as a genital structure can make it a likely target for symptoms when a patient's guilt is sexual in origin. Is a psychiatrist needed in these situations? I don't really think so unless it is felt that the special training and insight a psychiatrist is able to bring to a clinical problem are necessary for the satisfactory solution of that problem.

In those few cases where a physician genuinely cannot be certain as to whether or not prostatic infection is present, or even in those cases where it is probable that no infection at all exists, I can't argue with a trial of a week or two of an appropriate antibiotic. The prolonged use of these potentially dangerous drugs, however, in the absence of any bona fide indications for them is to be strongly condemned.

When the bacterial localization tests suggest the absence of any infection, as is usually the case in my experience, a detailed sexual history obtained from a patient will often reveal the fact that at about the time his symptoms started a change in his sexual habits occurred, which could directly be related to his symptoms. Marital disharmony, a recent onset of inability to achieve erections sufficient for intercourse, inability of a wife to have sexual relations because of problems with her own health, illness of a child in the family, and many other factors can combine to alter a man's usual ejaculatory pattern and to not infrequently lead to the condition of nonbacterial prostatitis (prostatostatis). This condition is, as we have seen, simply an accumulation of prostatic fluid within the prostate gland caused by a sudden decrease in the frequency of ejaculation. This problem is particularly acute for those men who feel that masturbation is not an acceptable substitute for intercourse, and so it is often these men who may develop the symptoms of nonbacterial prostatitis. Inasmuch as this condition is not a disease or an infection in a genital structure, patients can quite readily deal with the problem. I have found that virtually all of a patient's anxiety can be relieved simply by explaining his problem to him and strongly reassuring him that he does *not* have an infection in his prostate and that his condition will *not* lead to other problems. Moreover, most patients are appreciative of the physician's prescription for treatment which consists of increased ejaculatory frequency, particularly if it is to be achieved via sexual intercourse!

Acute Bacterial Prostatitis

Acute bacterial prostatitis is a very uncommon condition that has not been discussed before because it is *not* confused with the other prostatic problems already discussed. It results from a sudden infusion of bacteria into the prostate gland, either by direct extension from an infection in the urethra (such as nonspecific urethritis) or, very occasionally, by a blood-borne spread of bacteria from an infection somewhere else in the body. Patients with acute bacterial prostatitis are quite sick, generally run a fever of 102° or higher, have the malaise and aches and pains that one often associates with flu, and often have low abdominal or low back pain. Since there is considerable swelling of the prostate gland caused by this infection, the inside size of the prostatic urethra may be decreased to the point of making voiding difficult or even impossible. On such occasions, temporary catheter drainage is necessary. On digital rectal examination the prostate is acutely tender and very painful and the midstream urine specimen will invariably show 50,000 to 100,000 colonies of bacteria per milliliter of urine. If there are no bacteria in the bladder urine, the diagnosis of acute bacterial prostatitis is highly unlikely. Making the correct diagnosis of this condition in the presence of urinary infection is not at all difficult. Treatment is by antibiotics, bed rest, and careful follow-up to minimize the likelihood of resulting chronic bacterial prostatitis.

In those patients whose symptoms are thought to be from acute bacterial prostatitis but in whom the urine culture is negative, and in those patients in whom acute bacterial prostatitis is *not* the diagnosis, other conditions which should be considered include acute appendicitis and renal colic (the passage of a kidney stone down the ureter and towards the bladder).

4

Benign Prostatic Hyperplasia (BPH)

WRT, a 57-year-old automobile salesman, made an appointment to see me recently. He told my nurse that it was nothing urgent, then canceled his appointment on two occasions over the next month before he finally showed up in my office. When I introduced myself to him, he assumed an apologetic air and told me that he had canceled the two appointments because he really hated to take up my time for what he was sure didn't amount to anything.

"Doc, I just don't understand it," he began. "I'm sure that there's nothing wrong with me. I'm in great shape, I exercise regularly, and I've never felt better." He paused, and then he added, "Maybe all I need is a pill or something. I dunno, it seems to take me forever to get my water started and I guess my stream isn't very strong, either."

I asked him how long he had these problems and he said that it had been about two or three years and he thought it was getting worse. He added that he had to get up two or three times at night to go to the bathroom.

"I guess what really bothers me most," he muttered, "is that when my stream finally starts, it just sort of stops pretty soon for a few seconds and starts again, and then when I think I am all done making water and I zip up my pants, more urine comes out and I wet myself."

I asked him to tell me a bit more about his delay in starting his urinary stream and also a bit more about just how weak his stream was.

"Well," he started, "when I feel like I've gotta go it just seems to take forever for me to start. I guess maybe it really isn't so long, though; maybe a half minute and even a minute. Heck," he shrugged, "it'll get better soon."

I asked him if he ever dribbled urine on the floor right around the toilet and he suddenly looked up at me and said, "How'd you know that? Yeah, that's exactly what happens and that's exactly how I know my stream isn't as good as it used to be. I have to stand right over the bowl now to keep from wetting the floor."

"And I'll bet that when you get an urge to make water," I said to him, "you've really got to go right away and pretty badly."

"Yep, I sure do, Doc. Is all this in my mind? I just can't imagine that anything could be wrong down there," he said, pointing to his genital area.

This patient demonstrated, with almost classic detail, the symptoms that usually accompany BPH, although many patients with this condition will not necessarily have every one of these symptoms.

Benign prostatic hyperplasia (BPH), sometimes referred to as benign prostatic hypertrophy, is a very common occurrence and is best thought of as a natural part of aging. Quite simply, it is a process in which the prostate gland enlarges. When the condition is present, however, there are not always symptoms of which the patient is aware; so there may be a considerable discrepancy between the actual existence of this condition and the frequency with which it produces symptoms. An analysis of autopsy studies reveals that over half of men who are 50 years of age or older and about three-quarters of men who are over 70 years of age actually have BPH. You should keep in mind, though, that this is an anatomic finding and reveals nothing whatever about the actual number of patients in whom these anatomic changes produce symptoms. A good estimate is that about one-quarter of these men who have the anatomic changes of BPH will also have the symptoms which will send them to their physician.

The cause of benign prostatic hyperplasia is poorly understood, although it is unquestionably related to the presence of circulating male hormones. Because of this, BPH is not found in eunuchs, for example, the very small percentage of males whose testicles were removed or became nonfunctioning prior to puberty. It is interesting to note that BPH seems in no way to be related to sexual activity, since it occurs in celibate priests with the same frequency that it occurs in the general male population. It is also not apparently related in any way to sexual excesses or deprivation at any time of life. Moreover, BPH as far as we know is not related to prior infection or inflammation of the prostate nor to cancer of the prostate (although prostate cancer and BPH can and do certainly coexist in the same individual).

The concept of BPH can be a difficult one to understand. I have found that a genuine comprehension of BPH can readily be achieved if the normal prostate gland is visualized as an apple with the core removed, as shown in Chapter 1 (see Fig. 1–2). The top of the apple (where the stem is) should be pictured fitting snugly against the bladder neck. The opposite end of the apple from the part with the stem may be seen to rest up against the membranous urethra, which is that part of the urethra within the sphincter muscle that a man contracts when he wants to suddenly shut off his stream of urine while voiding (Fig. 4–1). The channel through the apple created by removing its core represents the prostatic urethra; it is through this channel that urine normally flows after leaving the bladder. This channel, the prostatic urethra, becomes obstructed when the prostate gland begins to enlarge, a process that usually begins around age 40 to 45 (Fig. 4–2). The prostatic urethra has a wall or lining just as any tubular structure in the body has a lining, and it is just beneath this lining that benign prostatic hyperplasia begins. This new growth of the prostate may occur most of the way or part of the way around the prostatic urethra—although it does not necessarily grow in a

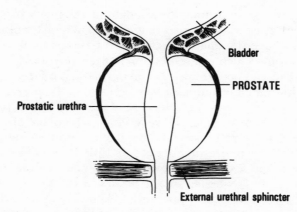

Figure 4–1   *The prostate gland and the external urethral sphincter. Note the relationship between the two. It is the external urethral sphincter which is contracted when a man wishes to shut off his urinary stream.*

Figure 4–2   *The prostate gland showing an early stage of benign prostatic hyperplasia (BPH). Note that this arises just underneath (outside) the lining of the prostatic urethra.*

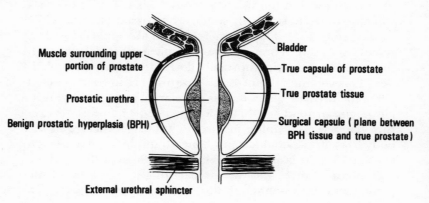

symmetrical manner. Therefore, there may be more new growth of the prostate on one side than on the other, or on the bottom (the floor) of the prostatic urethra rather than on either side. This new growth is made of the same types of tissue as the normal prostate gland although in different proportions. The normal prostate gland is made up of fibrous or connective tissue, muscle, and glands (see Chapter 1); the new growth of prostate will have the same tissues but will usually have more fibrous and muscular tissue. As the growth of new prostate tissue (BPH) slowly continues, which it does inexorably over a long period of time usually measured in years, it tends to grow in an outward as well as an inward direction (Fig. 4–3). When it grows toward the outside of the prostate gland it tends to compress the true, normal prostate tissue between itself and the true capsule of the prostate gland (the skin of the apple). The point where the expanding new growth of prostate (the BPH) meets the normal and true prostate tissue is called the surgical capsule. During surgery for BPH, it is only the new growth of BPH tissue that is removed (see Chapter 6). When this new BPH tissue grows towards the outside of the prostate gland, it can be felt as an enlarged prostate on digital rectal examination. However, an outward growth of the new prostate has nothing to do with bringing about any of the symptoms that a patient would notice and that are associated with BPH. Usually, though, if the new prostate tissue grows in an outward direction it also will grow in an inward direction. This will decrease the inside size of the prostatic urethra. It is the narrowing of this channel through which the urine flows that produces the characteristic symptoms associated with benign prostatic hyperplasia (Fig. 4–4).

It is important for a patient to understand that only three parts or lobes of the prostate (out of five) can cause the symptoms of BPH. These are the two lateral lobes and the middle lobe. The two lateral lobes can be felt on digital rectal examination (Fig. 4–5) if they enlarge in an outward direction; but the middle lobe can never, under any circumstances, be felt because it is enlarging into the channel of the prostatic urethra from the floor of that urethra. This middle lobe growing up from the floor can be thought of as if the *lower* half of the

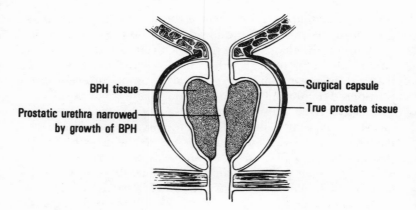

Figure 4–3   *The prostate gland showing considerable growth of benign prostatic hyperplasia. Note how it encroaches upon and pushes into the channel of the prostatic urethra.*

Figure 4–4   *The prostate gland showing a severe degree of benign prostatic hyperplasia that almost totally replaces the true prostate tissue by compressing it peripherally against the true capsule of the prostate. Note particularly how the benign prostatic hyperplasia also grows in an inward direction, virtually obliterating the channel of the prostatic urethra through which urine must pass.*

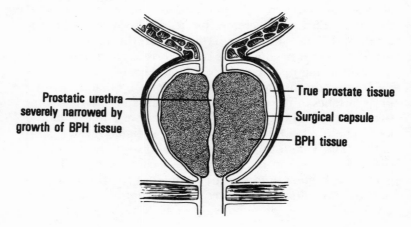

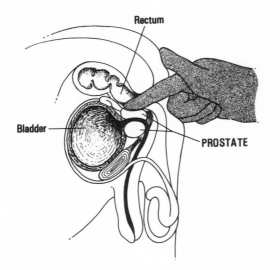

A

Figure 4–5   Digital rectal examination of the prostate gland.
A. A lateral view of the examining finger palpating the prostate gland.
B. A view from straight overhead as if the patient were bent over sharply at the waist and you are looking down from the ceiling.

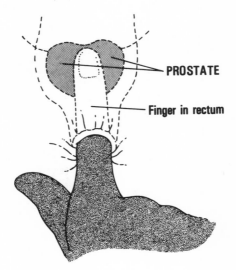

B

apple produced a growth of BPH directly into its core while the examining finger, when placed in the rectum, is only able to feel the *upper* half of the apple. Therefore, when a rectal examination is done (Fig. 4–6) to ascertain whether the prostate is "enlarged," the only parts of the prostate that can be felt and that can be causative of the symptoms of BPH are the lateral lobes. *The middle lobe, never palpable, is probably the most common cause of the symptoms of BPH.*

Effects of BPH on the Bladder

If the process by which the new growth of prostatic tissue results in a partial or complete blockage of the channel through which the urine must flow is understood, it is relatively easy

Figure 4–6   *A digital rectal examination of the prostate. Note how it is absolutely impossible for the examining finger to palpate the middle lobe of the prostate gland even though it might be severely enlarged and obstructing the flow of urine.*

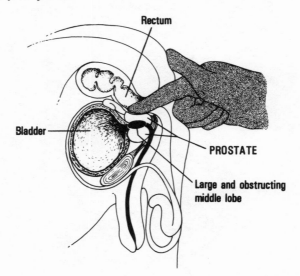

Rectum

Bladder

PROSTATE

Large and obstructing middle lobe

to then recognize and comprehend the symptoms that accompany this process. The act of voiding is the contraction of the bladder muscle on the one hand and the resistance to the flow of urine on the other. The channel through which the urine flows once it leaves the bladder is really just a tube that runs from the neck of the bladder all the way to the opening on the very end of the penis. Whenever anything encroaches upon the interior dimensions of the tube, such as the growth of new prostate tissue, the bladder muscle has to work harder in order to carry out its mission of emptying itself during voiding. Under normal circumstances, there should be no urine left in the bladder following voiding. Bladder muscle, though perhaps more complex in its structure than most muscles in the body, will nevertheless react like any other muscle to hard work. When the bladder has to contract more forcefully in order to empty itself because of an increased resistance to the flow of urine caused by an enlarged new growth of prostate, the bladder muscle undergoes a buildup and a strengthening in much the same manner that the upper arm and chest muscles enlarge and build up when a man begins a vigorous exercise program that includes pushups. Because of the unique nature of bladder muscle, the buildup that the bladder undergoes is an irregular one; it is not uniform throughout and generally begins in the trigone of the bladder, that part of the bladder just inside the bladder neck and on the floor of the bladder.

As the obstruction to the flow of urine becomes progressively more severe over a period of months or years, the muscle buildup within the entire bladder, including the trigone, continues so that the bladder will have enough strength to empty itself during voiding. The increased muscle buildup on the trigone results in daytime voiding frequency in addition to nocturia. As long as the bladder muscle is able to build up to the point that it can overcome the resistance offered by the slowly enlarging prostate gland it will be able to empty itself during voiding; the bladder in this condition is said to be compensated.

The new growth of BPH tissue into the channel of the prostatic urethra and the resulting obstruction to the flow of urine is invariably a progressive phenomenon, albeit a very slow one, that proceeds over a period of months to years. As the obstructive process continues, the buildup of bladder muscle produces an irregular appearance known as bladder trabeculation (Fig. 4–7). Trabeculation is characterized by irregular bands of muscle that have built up within the bladder; the areas between these built-up muscle bands are recessed or "popped out" much like a Mickey Mouse balloon in which the nose and the ears "pop out" as you continue to blow into the balloon. These "pop-out" areas are called cellules; they are not nearly as deep as the "pop-outs" in the Mickey Mouse balloon but they are several millimeters and even up to a centimeter in depth and they are recessed back from the thickened and built-up muscle bands. In extreme and long-standing cases of obstruction caused by BPH, these cellules can indeed pop out for several centimeters; they are then called diverticulae.

Symptoms of BPH

The trigone of the bladder is located just inside the bladder neck, on the floor of the bladder, so that urine comes in contact with it before any other part of the bladder. Because of its very dependent position, even small amounts of urine can cover the trigone when other parts of the bladder are not yet in contact with urine. The trigone is the most sensitive part of the bladder, and when urine comes in contact with it the urge to void is transmitted from the bladder to the brain. It has already been noted that the trigone is the first part of the bladder to undergo the muscle buildup that results from obstruction to the flow of urine, and it is this muscle buildup that results in the increased sensitivity of the trigone to the presence of much smaller than normal amounts of urine.

The first actual symptom that results from BPH is due to this heightened sensitivity of the trigone: an increase in the frequency of the desire to void. This is initially perceived as an increase in the number of times a man is awakened at night by a voiding urge after he has gone to sleep. This symptom is know as nocturia (it should be noted that the term is not

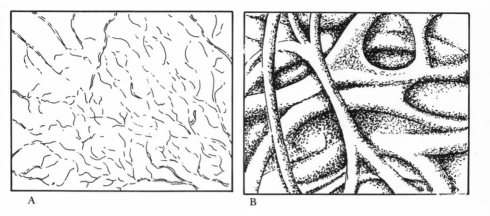

A

B

Figure 4–7   A. *The interior of a normal bladder. Note the very smooth appearance of the bladder wall. The little lines indicate the normal presence of blood vessels which are just underneath the bladder lining and are readily visible when viewed through a cystoscope.*

B. The inside of the bladder showing the buildup of the bladder muscle (trabeculation). This buildup of the bladder muscle can become so severe that areas between the built-up strands of muscle actually "pop out" and form little outpouchings known as "cellules."

C. A normal cystogram. Note the perfectly normal, smooth, and regular outline of the bladder.

D. A cystogram of a person with severe bladder outlet obstruction due to BPH. Note the marked irregularity of the bladder outline caused by the pronounced muscle buildup of the bladder wall (trabeculation) and by the numerous outpouchings (cellules) related to this muscle buildup. The shadow in the center of the bladder is caused by a very enlarged middle lobe of the prostate gland.

C   D

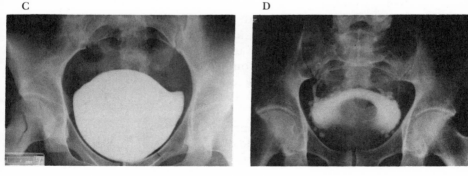

applicable if a man is awake during the night for other reasons, and while in that sleepless condition he decides to void). As a general rule, approximately five ounces (150 cc) of urine are present in the bladder before a voiding desire is apparent, but during conditions of sleep something more than this amount is normally required before a person will be awakened. It is the increased irritability of the trigone due to its muscle buildup that triggers a voiding urge strong enough to awaken a man even though there is considerably less urine present in the bladder than would otherwise be required to awaken him. During waking hours, the kidneys generally make approximately two ounces of urine (60 cc) each hour, but during sleep the urine output is decreased so that most individuals can normally go for a full eight hours of sleep without being awakened to void. With the muscle buildup of the trigone and its resulting increased irritability, however, men will awaken to void once, twice, or even three, four, or five times per night. And once nocturia begins it invariably becomes more pronounced with the passage of time.

You may wonder why the muscle buildup of the trigone results in a man having to get up at night to void (nocturia) and not in an increased frequency of daytime voiding. The answer is that there usually is a daytime frequency that results as well, but when people are up and around and busy doing things the voiding urge is usually not perceived very strongly in its initial stages and is frequently ignored until it becomes more pronounced. During sleep, however, there is nothing else distracting the brain and voiding urges are perceived strongly both early and often. Even the dreams that people sometimes have in no way detract from the voiding urge that awakens them. In addition to the symptoms of nocturia and frequency, the problem of urgency also is a fairly common one relatively early in the course of BPH. It also is caused by the muscle buildup and increased sensitivity of the trigone. Urgency can best be defined as "when you have to go, you have to go *right now*."

The bladder, alas, can only continue its muscle buildup to a certain point in its efforts to overcome the obstruction caused by the growth of new prostate tissue. But the obstruction itself usually progresses inexorably, so a patient sooner or later begins to perceive the symptoms of hesitancy and a weak urinary stream. Hesitancy is the term used when a man has to stand at the urinal for anywhere from several seconds to a couple of minutes waiting for the urine flow to start while the bladder muscle strains against the significant resistance caused by the new growth of prostate. Eventually the flow of urine starts but the stream is weak and not particularly forceful, an occurrence particularly troublesome when a man has to void after he has allowed his bladder to get overstretched as might happen, for example, during a long car trip or a good movie. An overstretched bladder that has gradually lost its tone over a period of months or years may not be able to contract at all or, much more commonly, it may contract only weakly and with great difficulty. It must be pointed out that this hesitancy in starting the urinary stream does *not* refer to the hesitancy that occurs when a man has difficulty initiating his stream while in a public restroom with many men lined up behind him waiting a turn at the urinal. This latter is an example of psychogenic hesitancy and is in no way related to benign prostatic hyperplasia.

As the obstructive process continues, the bladder eventually is not able to empty itself during the contraction that normally occurs with voiding, and so a patient may observe the symptom of intermittency. This means that the urinary stream stops before the completion of voiding and some seconds later it starts again. This is caused by the inability of the bladder to empty itself completely on one contraction, thereby requiring a second and weaker contraction of the bladder which occurs after a very brief recuperative period for the bladder muscle. Sometimes this intermittency occurs very near the end of the urinary stream when the patient thinks that he is quite through voiding; anywhere from a small amount to an ounce or more of urine may be expelled by the second and weaker bladder contraction after the patient has already closed his trousers. This is known as terminal dribbling and is a fairly common complaint among sufferers of BPH. It should not be confused with the few drops of urine that commonly escape from the end of the penis when they become trapped in the prostatic urethra during a hasty termination of voiding. Those few drops of urine then leak out subsequent to closing the trousers, completely unrelated to BPH, when the external sphincter muscle relaxes.

Eventually, the bladder that is obstructed by the BPH reaches the point where it can no longer empty, even with a second contraction; at this point the bladder becomes a decompensated one. This means that some residual urine is present after voiding; the amount of this residual urine can be very accurately measured by catheterizing or cystoscoping the patient immediately after voiding and noting the amount of urine that returns through the catheter or through the inside of the cystoscope. Normally, there should be no residual urine after voiding. Alternatively, the amount of residual urine can be estimated on the post-voiding x-ray film that is taken as a part of an excretory urogram or by an abdominal ultrasound exam, but these methods are not as precise as the other two methods. When a bladder has become a decompensated one, the amount of residual urine will initially be minimal but will invariably increase with the passage of time. It is not at all unusual to have a pint or even a quart of urine left in the bladder following voiding in advanced cases of bladder outlet obstruction due to BPH. I do not get too concerned about the amount of residual urine until there are three or more ounces of urine remaining in the bladder following voiding. It must be emphasized, however, that once residual urine is present following voiding it is usually only a matter of time before the amount of the residual urine increases greatly.

With the onset of residual urine, which is by definition a late occurrence in the BPH disease process, an additional set of symptoms may be anticipated. Once the residual urine has reached three or four ounces, the patient will notice that it is only a short time after voiding that he feels the need to void again. For example, if a patient leaves four ounces of urine behind following voiding, it would take only another ounce or two or perhaps three before he again feels the urge to void. This means that he may be voiding every thirty minutes to two hours. Frequency then, although present relatively early after the onset of BPH because of the buildup of muscle in the trigone, returns with the advent of residual urine and can become an even more significant problem to the patient. As the residual bladder urine builds up and increases to a pint or more, there may be no room left in the bladder for freshly made urine coming down from the kidneys. An involuntary leakage of urine out of the urethra may then result. This kind of incontinence is known as overflow or paradoxical incontinence, and it is not an uncommon finding with advanced bladder outlet obstruction due to BPH. As a matter of fact, I feel quite strongly that whenever a man over 40 has an involuntary leakage of urine, usually occurring during sleep but often a daytime occurrence, bladder outlet obstruction due to BPH with overflow incontinence is far and away the most likely explanation for the problem.

Once the bladder has decompensated and residual urine has become a reality, infection in the bladder may well occur before too long. This is because urine is an almost ideal fluid for nurturing the growth of bacteria which may originate in various portions of the urethra or in the prostate gland. These bacteria have most probably been totally asymptomatic and have caused no prior difficulty; but when given a large pool of stagnant urine in which to grow, there is often rapid multiplication of the bacteria until a symptomatic infection exists. If a bacterial infection in the bladder occurs, the patient will notice an acute worsening of his symptoms of frequency and urgency and the urine will not infrequently have a foul or "stable-like" odor caused by the release of ammonia resulting from the action of certain kinds of bacteria on the urine itself. The action of these bacteria tends to make the urine highly alkaline and this, in turn, can lead to the precipitation of stones in the bladder. These stones can produce relatively few symptoms but can also be the cause of severe pain and discomfort.

Hematuria (blood in the urine), visible either to the naked eye or when the urine is examined under a microscope, is a fairly common occurrence with benign prostatic hyperplasia. Indeed, BPH represents one of the two most common causes of hematuria in men over 40 (with bladder cancer the other). The blood vessels supplying the urethra and bladder neck travel in the tissue just underneath their lining, and this is the precise area where the BPH tissue grows. As it grows, BPH tissue stretches the blood vessels that lie on top of it; this stretching can ultimately lead to a bursting of these blood vessels. If a very small blood vessel bursts, the hematuria will be seen only microscopically; if a larger blood vessel bursts, the hematuria will be seen with the naked eye as pink or red urine. Severe hemorrhage from this source is a very uncommon occurrence, but it does happen and is one indication for the surgical removal of the obstructing (and bleeding) prostatic tissue.

As the new growth of obstructing BPH tissue continues to enlarge and to produce more symptoms of increasing severity most patients will eventually visit a physician to seek an understanding and a resolution of the problem. A small and interesting minority of patients, however, are seemingly unaware of any voiding difficulties and therefore do not seek medical help. For these individuals the natural history of their disease may follow one of two routes. The first route is a progression of the symptoms of obstruction until the time comes, suddenly and without warning, when the patient has the severe discomfort of acute urinary retention and is unable to pass any urine at all. Prompt treatment of this condition requires the passage of a catheter into the bladder in order to drain the urine. When one of these episodes of acute urinary retention occurs, the "handwriting is on the wall" and the patient will inevitably require surgical relief from his disease, surgery which should be done as soon as is convenient. The second and far more serious route that BPH may infrequently follow is that of kidney failure, uremic poisoning, and death. Once the bladder has become decompensated, the residual urine that remains after voiding invariably builds up to larger and larger quantities; in this small group of patients, the drainage of urine from the kidneys is blocked because the large amount of urine already present in the bladder prevents any more urine from entering. The high pressure in the bladder resulting from the great quantity of urine in it is transmitted back up to the kidneys where normal kidney function, which is to filter blood and thereby remove various waste products, is severely impaired. Uremic poisoning, which results when these various waste products are not filtered and removed by the kidneys, sets in and can be diagnosed by measuring the blood levels of creatinine and urea nitrogen, two of the waste products that must be removed (see Chapter 2). If satisfactory drainage of the bladder (and therefore of the kidneys) is not brought about promptly, coma and death will ensue.

A most interesting question that is usually asked is: Why and how is it possible for an individual who has BPH severe enough to lead to acute urinary retention or even death to not be aware of the symptoms of BPH at a much earlier stage that would have led him to a physician for help? I feel that there are three possible explanations for this seemingly extraordinary fact. First, the symptoms of bladder outlet obstruction (BPH) can be subtle in their onset and are usually very slow in their progression. It is therefore certainly a possibility that a patient gets so accustomed to his symptoms of bladder outlet obstruction that he cannot remember when he did *not* have them. Thus he considers the symptoms to be normal for him, thereby not requiring a visit to his physician. Second, since many men regard the prostate as a genital structure, and nothing is more important to them than their genitals—perhaps even life itself—these men are subconsciously unwilling to admit that they have any symptoms of prostatic disease and consciously completely deny all symptoms associated with the prostate gland. The patient cited at the beginning of this chapter, for example, certainly had a problem with disease denial, although not to the degree where he failed to seek medical help. Third, and a real consideration for many of limited financial means who have not been brought up in the mainstream of society, is that entry into the health care system is a foreboding process, a costly one, and one that is to be avoided if at all possible. For these individuals the symptoms of bladder outlet obstruction often represent nothing more than additional problems to the many already present in their troubled lives and just are not severe enough to warrant a physician visit.

Overall, I estimate that the vast majority of patients ultimately coming to surgery for BPH do indeed come to the physician because of one or more of the symptoms already noted. A small percentage of patients, perhaps 5 percent or fewer of those with BPH, will present themselves initially to a physician or an emergency room with the problem of either an inability to void (acute urinary retention) or the problems associated with uremic poisoning, which generally are those of severe weakness and fatigue.

Physical Examination

Your doctor will very probably begin by feeling your lower abdomen in order to detect whether your bladder is full. This is because one of the eventual occurrences with BPH is residual urine, and residual urine, once present, inevitably builds up to a large amount that can be detected by distention of the bladder. In very unusual circumstances a full bladder may reach all the way to the umbilicus, but it is not uncommon to find a bladder that is enlarged to a point halfway between the pubic hair and the umbilicus. This will happen with a patient who is not able to empty his bladder on voiding and carries 300 to 500 cc of urine as residual urine.

Digital rectal examination of the prostate gland is really the only other part of the physical examination that is germane to the diagnosis of BPH, although it must again be emphasized that it is certainly *not* a definitive examination since it cannot unequivocally determine if a patient does or does not have BPH. Even more importantly, it cannot reveal whether any BPH that *may* be present is actually producing obstruction to the flow of urine. This is because, as we have seen, it is often the middle lobe of the prostate gland that is most likely to produce symptoms of bladder outlet obstruction, and the middle lobe is *never* palpable on rectal examination. The lateral lobes of the prostate gland, on the other hand, are readily palpable on digital rectal examination, but enlargement of these lobes is only suggestive, and certainly not diagnostic, of obstruction to the flow of urine. As a general rule, if the lateral lobes are enlarged in an outward direction so that they feel enlarged to the examining finger, the chances are good that these same lateral lobes will also be enlarged in an inward direction and will encroach upon the channel of the prostatic urethra where they may or may not then produce symptoms of obstruction to the flow of urine. An equally general rule is that if the lateral lobes are not outwardly enlarged on digital rectal palpation they probably are not enlarged in an inward direction either. It should be clear, therefore, that the prostate gland that is only minimally enlarged or not enlarged at all tells the examining physician absolutely nothing about whether or not there is any middle lobe enlargement that could be quite significant; further, enlargement of the lateral lobes is suggestive but by no means conclusive that lateral lobe obstruction to the flow of urine might exist; finally, lateral lobes that are not enlarged on digital rectal examination suggest the absence of any lateral lobe obstruction to the flow of urine. In addition to the two lateral lobes, the posterior lobe is the only other lobe of the prostate that is palpable on rectal examination and this lobe is never a participant in the process of BPH.

I believe that the most important information to be gained from the digital rectal exam is probably that of whether or not the patient's prostate gland is suggestive of malignancy or is probably benign.

Diagnostic Studies
for Symptomatic Benign
Prostatic Hyperplasia

Urine Analysis and Urine Culture

The urine analysis is a standard part of the examination of any patient known or thought to have BPH. Even though this test does not directly contribute to the diagnosis of this condition, it is important for a physician to know if the patient has more than a very few white blood cells (pus cells) in the urine since this would suggest, but certainly not prove, the presence of a urinary tract infection. Also, it is important to know if there are any red blood cells in the urine (microhematuria) since the presence of blood in the urine pretty well mandates that kidney x-rays (an excretory urogram) be obtained prior to any possible prostate surgery. Although red blood cells are a common finding with BPH, they also can be a warning of serious disease in the kidneys or bladder which could be detected by the excretory urogram. Examination of the urine can reveal other important things about the general state of a patient's health such as the presence of sugar or protein in the urine (both abnormal) or the presence of white blood cells or bacteria in the urine (see Chapter 2). Besides the urine analysis, which can only suggest the presence or absence of infection in the urine, a urine culture may be indicated. A urine culture can document with certainty the presence of an infection. Should one be present, it must be treated promptly. Infection provides another strong indication for considering prostate surgery in a patient.

Blood Studies

There are no available blood studies that will diagnose benign prostatic hyperplasia; however, several studies are generally carried out during the course of a patient's evaluation for BPH, and they are virtually always done prior to any contemplated prostate surgery. One of these determinations is a blood creatinine level, since this is one of the best and certainly the simplest method for evaluating how well a patient's kidneys are functioning. An abnormal elevation of the creatinine level may be important for two reasons: first, it may represent a valid reason all by itself to consider prostate surgery in order to restore normal kidney function; second, any contemplated prostate surgery is best deferred until kidney function has been improved to its optimum, usually by means of prolonged catheter drainage. It is not at all unusual in some patients with BPH, when there has been a large amount of residual urine present for a prolonged period of time, to find an abnormal elevation of the blood creatinine level. This usually means that a patient has already suffered renal damage from back pressure on the kidneys. Such an elevation of the creatinine level does not necessarily mean that a patient is too sick for surgery, but it does mean that surgery should ideally be deferred until the kidney function has improved.

The other blood studies that are sometimes done when a patient is being evaluated for BPH or when prostate surgery is contemplated are acid and alkaline phosphatase levels and the prostate specific antigen level. Mild elevation of the prostate specific antigen (PSA) is seen with BPH but always requires further evaluation. High levels of PSA usually indicate the presence of prostate cancer. The alkaline phosphatase level, if elevated, suggests the possibility that the carcinoma has spread to the bone. While neither of these findings, if positive, would alter the requirement to treat the patient's symptoms of bladder outlet obstruction, the knowledge that a patient has prostate carcinoma may well modify the surgical approach or even the timing of the surgery (see Chapter 6). Elevation of the prostatic fraction of acid phosphatase is strong evidence not only of the presence of prostate cancer but also of its spread beyond the prostate gland itself.

X-ray and Other Imaging Studies

As a general rule, I like to get an excretory urogram in those patients thought to have BPH because it affords an opportunity to visualize and evaluate both the upper (kidneys and ureters) and lower (bladder and urethra) urinary tracts. The excretory urogram can assure me that my patient's kidneys are perfectly normal in appearance without any stones, tumors, obstructions, or other abnormalities that are best discovered before surgery. Moreover, since bladder x-rays are taken following voiding as a routine part of the excretory urogram, it is possible to get a very good estimate of how well a patient empties his bladder and how much residual urine is present in the bladder following voiding. The lower urinary tract can also be evaluated for bladder stones that may result from bladder infection caused by BPH. Finally, an excretory urogram is useful for estimating the size of the prostate enlargement (Fig. 4–8).

Although most urologists obtain an excretory urogram during the course of the preoperative evaluation and study of the patient with BPH, others avoid these x-rays and instead

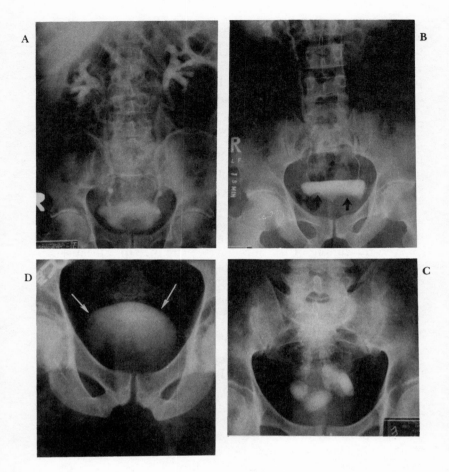

Figure 4–8 EXCRETORY UROGRAMS *(from different patients) demonstrating some of the abnormalities associated with benign prostatic hyperplasia. Compare these with a normal excretory urogram in Figure 2–1.*

A. Obstructed upper urinary tracts (kidneys and ureters) caused by BPH.

B. A marked elevation of the base of the bladder (arrows) caused by enlarged lateral lobes of the prostate (BPH).

C. Multiple stones within the bladder caused by high residual urine with resulting infection in the bladder. This film is taken prior to injection of the dye.

D. High residual urine seen on the post-voiding film. The inability to empty the bladder is caused by the large and obstructing prostate; the arrows indicate the outline of the enlarged bladder that is filled with contrast medium.

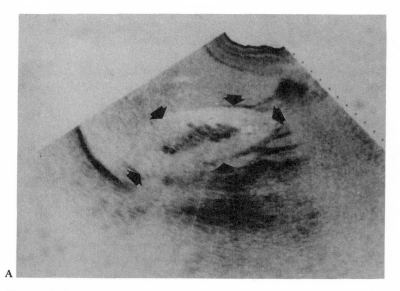

A

Figure 4–9 ULTRASOUND OF THE KIDNEYS.

   A. A perfectly normal kidney identified by the arrows.

   B. An obstructed kidney with dilation of the collecting system of the kidney caused by an enlarged prostate with back pressure on the kidney. Arrows identify the dilated collecting system of the kidney.

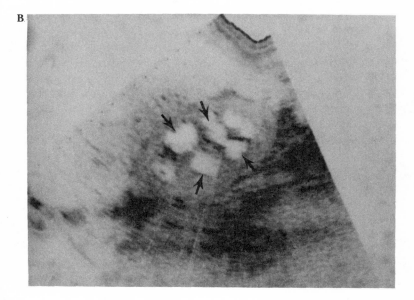

B

study the kidneys by means of ultrasound (Fig. 4–9) and kidney scans (Fig. 4–10). The combination of these two studies can admirably reveal almost everything that can be learned from an excretory urogram about the condition of the kidneys. Moreover, the quantity of residual urine can also be determined by scanning the bladder after the kidneys are scanned. The one strong indication for doing an excretory urogram and not the alternative techniques is when a patient has microscopic or visible hematuria that brings up the possibility of a small kidney tumor that might not be detected except by an excretory urogram.

Figure 4–10 RENAL SCAN.
Marked obstruction and enlargement of the kidney on the left caused by an enlarged and obstructing prostate gland. In the photograph on the left, note that the left kidney remains very dense over a progressive time interval as the injected radioisotope remains in the kidney and cannot drain out because of the obstruction. In the photograph on the right, an injection of a diuretic (a substance that makes the kidneys produce more urine) has been given to the patient and this serves to exaggerate even more the blockage to the left kidney. Note also the obstruction and dilation of the left ureter (the tube that drains the kidney). For comparison with a normal renal scan, see Figure 2–2.

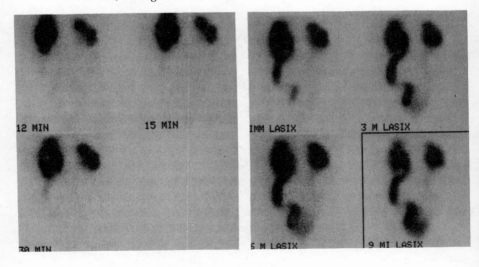

Urodynamic Studies

As noted in Chapter 2, urodynamic studies provide a reasonably accurate and reproducible means of determining quantitatively how efficiently the bladder is carrying out its two basic functions: urine storage and urine evacuation. The various urodynamic studies assess the function of both the bladder and the urinary sphincters, and it is possible to obtain several different measurements that, taken collectively, enable a physician to determine with accuracy the reason for a given patient's voiding difficulties. When these difficulties are those of obstruction due to BPH, they result from the increased resistance in the prostatic urethra to the flow of urine; the specific urodynamic study that is used to measure this is the urinary flow rate. This is the simplest of the urodynamic investigations and it is a measurement of the rate of urine flow, in milliliters per second, once an individual's maximum flow rate has been reached. In order for this test to be a valid one, a patient must have a bladder that is full enough to provide a good voiding urge; this usually means that the voided volume should be at least 150–200 ml. Once the stream of urine has reached what the patient feels is his maximum flow, the rate of that flow is then measured and compared with established norms. Men under 40 years of age should have a urinary flow rate greater than 22 ml/second; between 40 and 60 years the flow rate should be greater than 18 ml/second; and males over 60 years of age should have a flow rate greater than 13 ml/second. As a general rule, the lower the rate of flow in a patient with BPH, the greater the need for surgical treatment of the BPH. Although an abnormally slow flow rate can occur without any bladder outlet obstruction if the patient has a poorly functioning bladder muscle, it is a fact that the relative frequency of this latter condition, as compared to BPH in men over 40, effectively means that a urine flow rate under 10–12 ml per second is almost always caused by bladder outlet obstruction and not by an abnormal bladder.

Urodynamic studies are not done by many urologists because they are usually not necessary in order to document the diagnosis of BPH. Regardless, I believe that these studies do indeed have a diagnostic place in certain situations, particularly those which are borderline or questionable as far as the necessity for surgery on the prostate, because a patient's symptoms may be few and/or the residual urine amount may be very minimal.

Cystoscopic Examination

The diagnosis of bladder outlet obstruction caused by benign prostatic hyperplasia can usually be made after a careful history is obtained from a patient; the history will invariably disclose many of the symptoms already noted. Physical examination is of minimal help in making or confirming the diagnosis unless a patient happens to have a palpably enlarged bladder with a large amount of residual urine in it, but this is not a common finding. The digital rectal examination of the prostate gland is always done, and may at times be helpful if the lateral lobes are significantly enlarged to palpation. However, it is not a major determinant in the ultimate diagnosis of bladder outlet obstruction due to BPH. The blood and urine tests certainly cannot diagnose BPH, and even the excretory urogram can only strongly suggest the existence of this condition by demonstrating a high residual urine or a "negative" shadow in the bladder portion of the x-ray caused by enlarged lobes of the prostate. Certainly the urine flow rate can suggest strongly the diagnosis of BPH as the cause of bladder outlet obstruction. By combining all of these studies and tests the physician can be quite comfortable with the diagnosis of BPH without the need to perform a cystoscopy.

Nevertheless, cystoscopy must be considered as the *sine qua non* for the definitive diagnosis of BPH because it actually enables a urologist to *see* the degree of obstruction caused by the enlarged lobes of the prostate, as well as any changes within the bladder that have been caused by this obstruction (trabeculation). Cystoscopy also enables a urologist to evaluate the bladder to be sure that it has no other significant diseases in it such as an unrelated cancer. Finally, it enables a urologist to estimate the size of the growth of obstructing prostatic tissue so as to determine the best surgical approach for removal of this tissue (see Chapter 6). Cystoscopy *cannot,* however, assess the degree of *functional* obstruction; that is, it cannot by itself tell a urologist whether a given patient requires surgery for BPH. It can confirm a urologist's opinion that the symptoms from which his patient suffers do indeed appear to be caused by BPH.

The timing of the cystoscopic exam will often vary from urologist to urologist. I prefer to do the cystoscopic examination as the very last test immediately prior to the contemplated surgery in those patients in whom the diagnosis of BPH has been established with reasonable certainty by the various other means already noted. On the other hand, I generally cystoscope, in the office, those patients in whom I feel that significant BPH is probably not present and surgical intervention is probably not needed. Cystoscopy in this latter group of patients is done mainly for the purpose of establishing a baseline image of the degree of obstruction in the prostatic urethra so as to advise the patient about the likelihood of his developing significant outlet obstruction in the future. It is also done to rule out other conditions which can cause symptoms similar to those produced by BPH.

Cystoscopic examination, done gently and after adequate local anesthesia has been instilled in the urethra, is very easily done in an office setting as a general rule. However, when it is to be performed before planned surgery, I prefer to wait until the patient has been hospitalized because it is easier to more accurately assess the size of the prostate (and therefore the surgical approach) when the patient is under spinal or general anesthesia. Finally, I feel that cystoscopic examination in the presence of significant residual urine is fraught with the possible danger of introducing infection into the bladder, something that can better be avoided or treated in a hospital setting.

Treatment for BPH

Indications for Surgery

Surgical procedures for the treatment of bladder outlet obstruction caused by BPH are indicated in two broad groups of conditions which I like to consider *subjective* and *objective*.

Subjective Indications for Surgery. These are the complaints and the symptoms as stated by the patient; they are said to be subjective because it is difficult for a physician to measure them in a quantitative manner. Symptoms are subjective because the producing stimuli will produce differing symptoms (or no symptoms at all) in different individuals. For example, when a patient says that he has a "weak urinary stream" or "trouble starting his stream" it must be obvious that what one person would call a weak urinary stream would not necessarily be weak to another. The perception of stimuli, therefore, will vary from person to person as will even the reporting of identical symptoms. The difference between a stoic individual and a hypochondriac is considerable, and while the vast majority of people are at neither of these extremes the great middle ground between them still leaves much room for differing reports. For these reasons, I will rarely tell a patient that prostatic surgery is indicated based *only* upon his symptoms. I much prefer to wait until the patient himself firmly requests that something be done surgically to relieve him of his symptoms. In my experience, patients who announce that they are ready for surgery invariably have better postoperative courses and better long-term results than those who are told that their symptoms require surgery. To sum up: for those patients in whom relief of symptoms is the *only* indication for surgery, I believe that "watchful waiting" is the best course to follow. This means that I watch the patient to make sure his renal function does not deteriorate and I wait for him to tell me if and when he wants the surgery.

One final word on the subject of symptoms and their relationship to needed prostate surgery. When a patient's *only* symptoms are irritative (frequency and urgency), and there are none of the objective indications for surgery present, I generally am loath to do any sort of surgery. This is because, in my experience, patients whose *only indication* for surgery consists of these irritative symptoms usually do not get a particularly good result from the surgery. Their symptoms usually persist. Since they were not really caused by any BPH, the surgical relief of any existing BPH will usually not change anything.

Objective Indications for Surgery. These are the indications that are measurable and not dependent upon a patient's interpretation. Moreover, they are precise and specific enough that several physicians seeing the same patient could agree on the findings. A high residual urine, for example, is something that can be accurately measured (in milliliters). A heavily trabeculated bladder is something that can be observed through a cystoscope or seen on x-ray. Recurrent bladder infections can be documented by bacterial culture of the patient's urine. Acute urinary retention or overflow incontinence are findings that can be agreed upon by anyone witnessing them. Any one of these findings would indicate to me the need for surgery; more than one finding indicates a greater need for surgery. Another objective indication for prostatic surgery which does not occur very often is heavy bleeding from spontaneous rupture of the blood vessels that have been stretched to the point of spontaneous bursting by the new growth of prostate. Usually, such bleeding stops spontaneously and the surgery can then be scheduled electively, hopefully before any recurrence of the bleeding. Sometimes, however, the bleeding does not stop by itself and can only be controlled by emergency prostate surgery.

To sum up, then, the objective indications for surgical intervention include the following: residual urine (generally over 100 ml), recurrent infection, bladder stones, decreasing kidney function (rising blood creatinine level), obstruction to the drainage of the kidneys, acute urinary retention, and overflow incontinence.

A word about residual urine. The larger the volume of residual urine, the greater the need for prostate surgery. Since residual urine is a late finding in the inexorable growth process of benign prostatic hyperplasia, it is fallacious to think that surgical intervention should not be contemplated until residual urine is present. On the other hand, when it is present, surgical intervention is probably mandatory, and the larger the volume of residual urine the greater the need for surgery.

Nonsurgical Treatment

As of this writing, there really is no noninvasive or non-surgical treatment for benign prostatic hyperplasia that is as successful as surgery. While it is true that oral estrogens will shrink the prostate gland sufficiently to relieve many of a patient's symptoms, the side effects are usually quite unacceptable. These include loss of erections, and growth and tenderness of the breasts. A drug that has been used, experimentally, to shrink the prostate is Leuprolide (Lupron), which is primarily used in easing the symptoms of prostate cancer (see Chapter 5). It reduces the testosterone in the body to castrate levels resulting in a shrinkage of the prostate, but its side effects are significant and its value, therefore, remains to be determined. Other drugs that effectively reduce the body's testosterone levels to near zero have been used experimentally to relieve the symptoms of BPH, and some of these drugs have produced a salutory effect. Thus far, however, these have all been accompanied by unacceptable side effects, primarily consisting of a loss of libido or erections or both.

Although not approved by the Food and Drug Administration, some physicians treat benign prostatic hyperplasia with one or more of several drugs that relax the smooth muscle surrounding the prostate. This may, in turn, result in a "relaxation" of the entire prostate gland such that it can expand slightly in an outward direction and thereby presumably allow the channel of the prostatic urethra to enlarge. By increasing the inside measurements of the prostatic urethra, the existing obstruction to the flow of urine is decreased and urine flow is enhanced. The drug that has been used most successfully is terazosin (Hytrin) for which FDA approval is anticipated by the end of 1993. Although some patients who have been placed on the drug have reported a subjective improvement in their symptoms of bladder outlet obstruction and have even had objective findings—such as an increased flow rate—to suggest benefit of the drug, long-term placebo-controlled studies are needed to determine how beneficial this and similar drugs really are. The side effects of weakness, dizziness, and somnolence can affect up to a fourth or more of patients taking the drug.

Finasteride (Proscar) is a new drug that was approved by the FDA in the summer of 1992 for the treatment of BPH. It works by blocking the conversion of testosterone to dihydro-testertone, a substance needed for the maintenance of BPH. Finasteride actually shrinks the prostate gland in most men, but only about 40 percent of patients taking it are able to achieve objective signs of improvement—increased flow rate, etc. Further, it usually takes an average of six or more months of medication before a patient sees the hoped-for improvement in his voiding symptoms. Nevertheless, Finasteride does represent a real breakthrough in the nonsurgical treatment of BPH, and the side effects of this drug are minimal (about 7 percent of men complain of loss of libido or erectile ability but this is reversible with cessation of therapy). It is my feeling that this drug and / or the terazosin (once it receives FDA approval) are best suited for the patient in whom all of the indications for surgery are subjective—in other words, they are for the relief of the patient's symptoms in the absence of objective indications for surgery (see above). A great deal of research is going on now to see what the long-term effects of Finasteride are and also to evaluate the combination of Finasteride and terazosin. Also, a large research effort is being organized to see if early use of Finasteride can prevent BPH. The future looks promising for ongoing research into new and better drugs to treat and even to prevent BPH. I do feel, however, that as of 1993 the surgical approach to the treatment of BPH remains the "gold standard."

Psychological Considerations

There is undoubtedly a great deal of anxiety, and at times even fear, connected with almost any kind of physical disease even if it does not involve surgery. When the required form of treatment *does* involve a surgical procedure, the anxiety and particularly the fear increase dramatically. Diseases of the prostate gland are of particularly great concern to most men, and if the disease requires a surgical treatment it can inspire fearful thoughts of a most unhappy nature. As with many things that provoke fear, it is the unknown, and the out-and-out myths and old wives' tales that are most to blame for such concerns and anxieties. I cannot stress strongly enough how very important it is for a thoughtful and caring physician to explain to his patient exactly what is involved in the surgical procedure to cure BPH, what the complications of the surgery may be, what the convalescence period is like, and, of the utmost importance, what does *not* happen to the patient and to his sex life.

A very common and extraordinarily widespread myth about prostate surgery is that once a man has had it his sex life is finished. This absolute falsehood is undoubtedly passed along in the locker rooms, bars, and late-night poker games wherever men congregate. There is no question about the fact that a patient undergoing surgery will do better and have a smoother convalescence if he is relatively free of anxieties and fears of any kind, but particularly those related to the surgery. When the surgery is for BPH, the common and often-expressed fears about "the end of my sex life" can be very effectively countered by the physician who will take the time and the interest to do so. Since so much of erectile dysfunction (impotence) is psychic in origin, it is probably accurate to say that the patient who goes into surgery feeling quite certain that he will be impotent as a result of the surgery will often be exactly that. The facts of the matter are that a patient's sexual abilities following BPH surgery will usually be precisely the same as they were before surgery, with the caveat that most patients having surgery for BPH are in their 60s and 70s and some will already have a greater or lesser degree of erectile dysfunction *prior* to the surgery. It is a very convenient and easy thing for a patient, following surgery, to blame his sexual problems on the operation itself rather than admit to himself that the problem is "his own fault." It is also not unlikely that an elderly male who has lost interest in having a sexual relationship with his wife will see fit to attribute this loss of interest to the surgery. It is very unusual for a sexually active and interested man to lose the ability to maintain this activity and interest as a result of the surgery. This is so whether the operation is done transurethrally or by one of the "open" surgical methods (see Chapter 6).

Positive reinforcement of these facts prior to surgery truly works wonders in alleviating patient concern about the ability to continue with his sex life after surgery. The urologic surgeon usually understands, perhaps far more than other surgeons, that patients who are having surgery on the prostate gland need to be given an opportunity to ventilate their fears and their concerns. For those patients who are uncomfortable about initiating these discussions the urologist himself will often bring up the subject and speak to the patient's concerns. It is my feeling that there are really many excellent urologists practicing in this country, and most of them are as caring and thoughtful about their patient's needs and anxieties as they are excellent in the actual performance of the surgical procedures. I believe that if you as a patient find yourself in the care of a urologist, however technically excellent he may be, who is less thoughtful and less caring about your worries and your anxieties than you would really like for him to be, it is only logical for you to ask your primary care physician to refer you to another urologist.

Results of Surgery

There are very few surgical procedures with which I am acquainted that bring about a more dramatic improvement in the quality of life for a patient than the surgery for BPH. Although there are certainly many surgical procedures which can bring about the same "cure" that prostatic surgery affords, there really are precious few other kinds of surgical procedures after which a patient almost immediately notices a dramatic resolution of the distressing symptoms which were present before surgery. If the operation for benign prostatic hyperplasia is carried out by a competent urologic surgeon, and if it was recommended appropriately and properly for one or more of the indications already noted, the patient may confidently expect an excellent result. It is my opinion that when the results are less than very good or excellent, it usually is the result of a marginal indication for surgery or an operative procedure that has not been carried out in the best possible manner.

If the operation has been done using the surgical approach through the penis (the transurethral approach) (see Figs. 6–1 and 6–2), the patient can anticipate that he will be up and out of bed on the day following surgery, and eating pretty much his regular diet. He will have a catheter in his bladder for three or four days after surgery, and the most pain or discomfort that he should have is that resulting from the presence of this catheter. This "pain," however, is more of an irritative discomfort rather than a true pain. Sometimes a patient will have painful spasms of the bladder while the catheter is in place. These are usually caused by the catheter tip and the balloon on the end of the catheter coming in contact with the highly sensitive trigone of the bladder. These bladder spasms may usually be controlled by means of belladonna and opium rectal suppositories which diminish and usually stop the bladder spasms. These suppositories work because they contain specific medications that act locally on the bladder to stop the spasms. A patient will usually leave the hospital about the third or fourth day after surgery and the catheter is usually removed the day before or on that same morning. Complete internal healing in the site of the surgical procedure can take up to three months or thereabouts, and during this period of time a patient may have varying degrees of voiding discomfort, usually consisting of mild urgency, frequency, nocturia, or any combination of these. Usually, however, the patient has almost no unpleasant symptoms by the end of the third or fourth week after surgery. By that time he is almost always voiding with a strength of urinary stream that has not been enjoyed since he was in his 20s and 30s!

When the surgical procedure is done via one of the "open" operative procedures (this is rather uncommon and is usually reserved for very large prostate glands), much that has been said in this section still remains true; however, the hospital convalescence is prolonged significantly and the patient will usually remain in the hospital four to five days longer than he would with the transurethral approach. Also, there is considerably more postoperative pain following an "open" operative procedure because the abdomen is cut and the operative field is exposed by going through the layers of the abdominal wall. Postoperative eating and ambulating are also usually delayed for two to three days when this "open" approach is used.

With any of the operative approaches to benign prostatic hyperplasia the mortality is less than one percent, and the deaths that do occur are a reflection of the fact that the vast majority of patients undergoing prostate surgery are in an elderly age group. The cause of death in these patients is usually a heart attack or a pulmonary embolus. It is extraordinarily rare for the operative procedure itself to result in death.

5

Cancer of the Prostate

I saw two patients recently whom I would like to tell you about. The first of these patients was fortunate; the second was not.

TAE, a 59-year-old Porsche mechanic, was referred to me by one of the best family medicine practitioners in town because of a "suspicious" area on his prostate gland. The patient told me that he had gone to his family doctor for a "routine" physical exam, and he had been told, following the digital rectal part of the exam, that there was a "bump" on his prostate gland. His PSA level was 5.9, slightly elevated above normal, which is 0–3.9 ng / ml. He went on to say that his doctor had told him to come to see me for my opinion about what to do next.

"Honest, doctor, I don't see what all the fuss is about," the patient said to me. "I don't have any pain, I pass my water like I did twenty years ago, and nothing hurts me."

I did a rectal examination and felt this man's prostate and there was indeed a nodule, about 1 cm in size, on the right side of the prostate gland. I told the patient that a biopsy was necessary, performed it, and it showed that the "suspicious" part of his prostate was indeed cancer. Why did I say earlier that this man was fortunate even though he was found to have cancer? I said it because he had his cancer discovered before it had spread, and surgical removal of the entire prostate should hopefully cure this man. He was indeed fortunate in having had a family physician who performed annual digital rectal examinations of the prostate and who promptly referred for consultation any finding that did not seem normal.

The second patient was CDS, a 60-year-old salesman who called my office for an appointment because of a "backache." He told my nurse that he thought he must have "kidney trouble" and therefore he thought that he should see a urologist.

As soon as he walked into my office he pointed to the middle of his low back and told me, "Doc, the pain in there is really getting to me! I have had it for about a month now, it's not getting any better, and there doesn't seem to be anything I can do to relieve it." He went on to say that he had assumed it was a kidney infection because his wife had once been told that she had a kidney infection when she had similar pain.

When I did a rectal examination of my patient's prostate gland I was not at all surprised to find that a good part of it was rock hard and strongly suggestive of cancer. Subsequent x-rays of his back confirmed my suspicion that his back pain was caused by the spread of his prostate cancer to the bones of his lower spine. The prostate was biopsied to prove the diagnosis of cancer and palliative treatment was recommended. This type of treatment, by definition, means that the patient's cancer has progressed beyond the point where cure can be anticipated and therapy is simply palliative. It is directed at making a patient as comfortable as possible and prolonging life as long as it still has a degree of quality.

Unhappily, this patient's story was not at all unusual. Perhaps a third of all prostate cancers are not discovered until they have spread beyond the point where there is any real probability of cure.

Incidence of Prostate Cancer

Prostatic cancer is a very common form of cancer, and, if skin cancers are excluded, prostate cancer is the most frequent malignancy occurring in men, accounting for about

132,000 new cases in 1993. Looking at the statistics from another point of view, about 25 percent of all nonskin cancers diagnosed in men are of prostatic origin, and about 15 percent of all the male cancer deaths are prostatic in origin. Overall, prostatic cancer is the second most common cause of cancer death in men after lung cancer, and about 36,000 men will die in 1993 from this disease. The obvious discrepancy between the incidence of prostatic cancer and the death rate from this cancer is a clear reflection of the fact that in many cases prostatic cancer is of a very low-grade malignancy, and men die *with* it rather than *from* it. It has been estimated that up to 30 percent of men in the United States over 50 years of age may have cancer of the prostate gland, and yet only a fraction of these men will succumb to this disease. The actual size, in cubic centimeters, of the prostate cancer in any given man, as well as the microscopic appearance of the tumor— whether it is of low-grade or high-grade malignancy—are the determinants of whether that carcinoma will act in a relatively benign way by spreading very slowly over many years, or whether it will act in a highly malignant fashion with rapid spread through the body in a matter of months or a very few years. Prostatic cancer is very uncommon in men under 50, but it then manifests itself with increasing frequency, reaching a peak in the over-75 age group when as many as 60 to 70 percent of all men may have this condition in one form or another, but usually in the relatively milder form of low-grade malignancy. Though many hypotheses and interesting observations have been made, the cause of prostate cancer remains unknown.

There has recently been much written in the lay and the medical press about the idea that many men with localized (stage A or B) prostate cancer do not need to have any treatment other than "watchful waiting" with regular examinations, including periodic PSA levels which may be of help in determining if the cancer is growing. This recent publicity has resulted because of the known fact that the great majority of men with prostate cancer do indeed die *with* it and not *from* it. Statistically, if great numbers of patients are included in a study, it is safe to say that prostate cancer will not be the cause of death for the majority of these patients. However, for any one given patient this just cannot be said. Cancer, by definition, grows. Whether it will grow fast enough to kill a given patient—or make his life miserable—before he dies of some other cause is an absolute unknown, although the patient's age at the time the cancer is diagnosed and his general health are obviously determining factors. My very general rule of thumb is that if the patient and I believe that he has an anticipated ten or more years of life, I will encourage him to have definitive therapy—that is, surgery or radiation. Other factors that I take into account in making my recommendation to the patient are his PSA level and the degree of malignancy (high or low) found at the time of the prostate biopsy. In general, I am a firm believer that cancer of any kind is better *outside* of the patient than within him, but I always present my patients with the option of "watchful waiting."

Anatomic Location

In Chapter 1, I pointed out that the healthy prostate in the young adult is about the size of a chestnut, and it generally begins to undergo a benign pattern of new growth (BPH) when a man is in his mid-40s. I also likened the prostate to an apple and noted that benign prostatic hyperplasia usually arises in the central part of the prostate gland just under the lining of the prostatic urethra. Carcinoma of the prostate, on the other hand, usually arises (about 80 percent of the time) in the peripheral or outer part of the gland, usually in the true prostate tissue and just under the true capsule of the prostate (the skin of the apple). Since the vast majority of prostate cancers arise so near to the outside of the gland, it is usually possible to feel them on digital rectal examination of the prostate, as a nodule or a firm or hard area (Fig. 5–1). About 20 percent of the time, however, the prostate cancer will arise deep within the gland; in these patients, of course, it is not possible to feel or to diagnose the cancer on digital rectal examination.

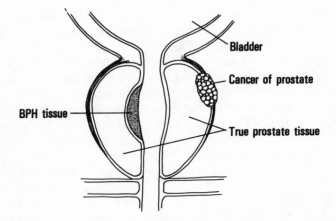

Figure 5–1   *The prostate gland with BPH and cancer. Note that, characteristically, BPH arises in the center of the gland, right around the prostatic urethra, and cancer arises in the periphery of the prostate where it can be palpated on digital rectal examination.*

Early and Late Symptoms
of Prostatic Cancer

Unfortunately, there are absolutely no symptoms of prostate cancer in its early stages. A possible exception to this statement might be a patient with a very rapidly growing and highly malignant prostate cancer with a rapid spread into the channel of the prostatic urethra so that early in the course of the cancer symptoms of bladder outlet obstruction would arise. Indeed, whenever an individual who has been voiding with no difficulty has a sudden onset of a very weak urinary stream with hesitancy, dribbling, intermittency, and perhaps incomplete bladder emptying, the presence of a rapidly growing carcinoma must be suspected. For this reason, I feel that these patients, who have symptoms of bladder outlet obstruction that have been present only for three to six months or less, should have a prostatic biopsy regardless of how the prostate may feel on digital rectal examination.

Much more frequently seen are patients with prostate cancer in whom the symptoms of bladder outlet obstruction do not come until very late in the course of the disease, after the diagnosis of cancer has been well established; the symptoms then result from the very slow growth of the cancer towards and into the prostatic urethra.

A common *late* finding of prostate cancer is the onset of pain in one or more bones that is constant and lasts for two weeks or longer. Such pain is most often in the spine although it may be in the bony pelvis, the low back, the hips, or the bones of the upper legs. When a patient with known prostatic cancer develops these pains, spread of cancer to the bone must be strongly suspected; when a patient over 50 who is not known to have cancer of the prostate comes to the doctor's office complaining of constant and severe pain in one or more of his bones, prostatic cancer with spread to bone should be considered in the physician's initial diagnostic approach. A digital rectal examination of the prostate should be carried out promptly to see if any areas suggestive of prostate cancer are noted, and bone x-rays, bone scans (see Chapter 2), and blood prostate specific antigen levels should also be done. Prostate biopsies are also necessary before any definite diagnosis of this disease can be made.

Making the Diagnosis of Prostatic Cancer

In the 80 percent of men in whom the prostatic cancer arises in the periphery of the prostate gland, the diagnosis of this condition may be suspected when a digital rectal examination of the prostate reveals a surface area that is something other than perfectly smooth and of uniform consistency. Areas on the prostate gland that feel nodular, irregular, or harder than the surrounding areas are not necessarily indicative of cancer, but they very definitely represent indications for a biopsy of that area and examination of the removed tissue by a competent surgical pathologist. The definitive diagnosis of prostatic cancer can be made only by the microscopic examination of removed prostate tissue. If prostatic cancer is to be diagnosed at a time when it is still curable, digital rectal examination of the prostate should probably be done annually in men over 50, and any suspicious prostate examinations should be referred promptly to a urologist for consultation and evaluation.

Obtaining Prostatic Tissue from Suspicious Areas

Since even the most "educated" examining finger will only be accurate about 50 percent of the time in differentiating benign from malignant lesions of the prostate, it is imperative that microscopic examination of the tissue from the suspicious area of the prostate be carried out, and this can only be done by means of a biopsy. I believe that the most accurate method for the diagnosis of prostate cancer uses ultrasound (see Chapter 2) to help guide the biopsy needle to that part of the prostate that is suspicious for cancer. This method certainly works and may be more sensitive in locating areas of cancer that cannot readily be identified with the examining finger. The serum prostate specific antigen (PSA) test comes close to being one of the best screening tests for cancer in medicine today. Even a slight elevation requires careful evaluation using a digital exam, a transrectal ultrasound exam, and possibly random prostate biopsies. The higher the PSA elevation the more likely the presence of cancer. This same test is also highly accurate in determining if a patient thought to be cured of cancer has suffered a recurrence of the cancer.

It must be emphasized again, however, that the prostate specific antigen is made by both normal and cancerous prostate cells. Therefore a large benign prostatic hyperplasia can cause an elevation of up to twice the normal levels of PSA. However, when the level of PSA is *more* than two to three times the upper limit of normal, prostate cancer must be strongly suspected.

Bone X-rays and Bone Scans

The role of bone x-rays and bone scans in prostatic cancer is simply to determine if there is any objective evidence that the cancer has spread to bone. In other words, bone scans and bone x-rays *only* play a role in the diagnostic study of those patients known to already have cancer of the prostate or those patients in whom cancer is strongly suspected but in whom the prostatic biopsies have been equivocal or perhaps have not been done for some reason.

When cancer of the prostate spreads beyond the confines of the prostate gland the prostate specific antigen blood level will usually but not always be elevated. Whether or not the PSA is elevated, if the patient is thought to be a candidate for curative surgery, every test must be carried out to be as certain as possible that the cancer has not spread beyond the confines of the prostate gland. This is because such spread might possibly place the patient beyond the hope of a cure and might therefore make pointless any contemplated surgery.

The two principal routes of spread of prostate cancer are to the lymph nodes of the pelvis deep within the body cavity, and to various bones of the body, primarily the spine, the pelvis, the hips, and the upper legs. There is no way to tell if the lymph nodes have cancer in them except by a direct surgical exploration of the nodes with a microscopic examination. However, spread to the bones can usually be detected by x-rays or bone scans, and the latter will reveal evidence of spread to bone several months before the bone x-rays develop their characteristic appearance (see Fig. 2–6). When cancer from the prostate spreads to bone there is usually an initial partial destruction of that bone followed by the body's normal reparative process which consists of a laying down of new bone in the area of the destruction. If the bone destruction is extensive, and the reparative process is not, the x-ray appearance of the affected bone will be one of rarefaction or thinning, which may make the bone look like it has punched-out lesions. If the bone destruction is not very extensive, then the reparative process will be the predominant x-ray finding, one of increased bone density. The former lesions are called lytic and the latter are known as blastic. Several months before metastatic spread of any kind to the bone is detectable by x-ray, bone scans are able to detect the process of regeneration and laying down of new bone in areas that have been the site of cancer spread.

Bone scans are made by injecting a radioactive material into an arm vein, which then concentrates in bone, and the amount of radioactive material that is taken up by each bone is accurately determined by a counting machine that scans the entire body. Wherever there has been destruction of bone there will be bone repair and regeneration, and wherever this occurs there will be an increased uptake of the radioactive material. The increased uptake of the isotope is detected by the counting machine and gives a dense appearance to the scan in those specific bones that are undergoing the reparative process (see Fig. 2–7). Whenever there is an increased radioactivity count over one or more bones it is strongly suggestive of cancer spread to those bones. However, there is a caveat: bone scans are not specific to the detection of cancer but only reflect the reparative process of bone. This process may also be found in response, for example, to bone fractures or even to arthritis. The increased uptake of radioactivity, though, in one or more bones in the presence of known cancer of the prostate is strongly suggestive that cancer spread has occurred, although actual biopsy of the bone to prove or disprove the presence of cancer is sometimes done. The correlation of bone scans and bone x-rays can often suggest whether an area of increased uptake in a bone is due to cancer spread or to something more benign, because the presence of an old fracture or any arthritic changes can usually be detected on bone x-ray. Because of this, bone biopsies are only rarely necessary.

For the patient known to have cancer of the prostate, then, the role of bone scans and bone x-rays is twofold: First, for the patient thought to have curable prostate cancer, because there is no evidence of spread anywhere beyond the confines of the prostate gland, bone x-rays and bone scans are carried out in the expectation that they too will be negative and to make sure that they are, in fact, negative. This use of bone scanning and bone x-rays is one of the steps in the process known as "*staging*" a patient to ascertain the presence or absence of cancer spread beyond the confines of the prostate gland.

Second, bone scans and bone x-rays "follow" patients with

known prostate cancer to see if and when additional spread of the disease occurs. Such patients may already have had an attempt at curative radical surgery (see Chapter 6), or they may be patients who have had radiation therapy in an attempt to cure them, or they may be patients who were seen for the first time when they were already beyond the point of cure. For each of these categories of patients, bone x-rays and bone scans at approximate yearly intervals are a means of observing and following the progress of these patients, not in the hope of curing them should the cancer appear in one or more bones, but to help predict the future course of their illness and to begin additional treatment as promptly as possible once the cancer spread has been determined. PSA determinations on a regular basis have replaced the need for yearly bone scans or bone x-rays in the opinion of many urologists. A rising PSA level, however, will often result in sending the patient for bone scans and / or bone x-rays.

Abdominal CT scans or an MRI with an endorectal coil can also be helpful in determining the presence of enlarged lymph nodes in the patient already diagnosed with prostate cancer. The presence of enlarged nodes might indicate spread of the tumor beyond the prostate gland itself, but both CT scans and use of the MRI are fraught with many false positives and false negatives and surgical removal of the pelvic lymph nodes, with microscopic examination of these nodes, is the only certain way of determining whether or not the prostate cancer has spread to these nodes.

Classification of Prostate Cancer

At the beginning of this chapter the statement was made that perhaps as many as 30 percent of men over age 50 have cancer of the prostate, but the vast majority of these men die *with* the disease and not *from* it. Certainly, every urologist can think of many patients alive and well five, ten, even twenty or more years after prostate cancer has been diagnosed. Unhappily, every urologist can also bring to mind a number of patients

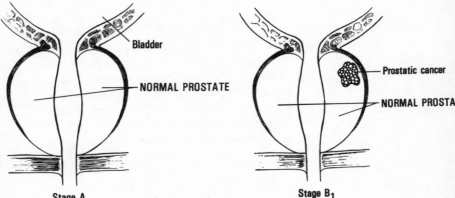

Figure 5–2 THE PROSTATE GLAND SHOWING THE DIFFERENT STAGES
OF CANCER.
   Stage A. *This is the "occult" stage of prostate cancer in which it cannot
be felt or detected in any way on digital rectal examination.*
   Stage B₁. *This is the stage where cancer is definitely palpable on digi-
tial rectal examination. It is smaller than one or two centimeters in size
and is localized to one side of the prostate gland.*

who lived for only a year or two after the diagnosis of prostate
cancer was made. Why the difference? Are there really such
things as "good" cancers and "bad" cancers?

   In an effort to answer these questions and to plan and
implement appropriate therapy for what seemed to be almost
two different diseases, retrospective studies of large numbers
of patients with prostate cancer were carried out. In these
studies, analyses were made of the size of the cancer at the
time of diagnosis (known as the "stage" of the prostate cancer)
and of the microscopic appearance of the cancer as to whether
it had the characteristics of low-grade or high-grade malignancy (known as the "grade" of the prostate cancer). These
two factors, size and microscopic appearance, were then studied and compared with the kind of treatment that the patient
received, whether there were any findings of spread of the
cancer, and perhaps, most importantly, how long the patient
lived after the diagnosis was made.

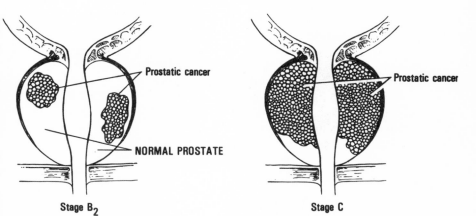

Stage B₂   Stage C

Stage B_2. *A more extensive form of cancer in which the cancer is larger than two centimeters or present on both sides of the prostate. B_1 and B_2 lesions can be detected on digital rectal examinations of the prostate gland.*

Stage C. *An extensive prostate cancer involving much of both sides of the prostate gland but where it is thought that the cancer has not spread outside of the prostate gland.*

There is no illustration for a stage D cancer because, by definition, a stage D cancer is one in which the prostate cancer has spread outside the confines of the prostate gland. A cancer that is originally thought to be a stage B or C can turn out to be a stage D. Even some of the occult A lesions can turn out to be stage D.

As a result of these very extensive studies, cancer of the prostate was classified into stages A, B, C, and D, with sub-classifications of the A, B, and D categories based upon the actual size, extent, and location of the cancer as well as its microscopic appearance at the time of diagnosis (Fig. 5–2).

Stage A is cancer that cannot be felt on digital rectal examination or suspected for any reason. It is diagnosed when a man has surgery for what is thought to be BPH and the pathologist reports the presence of cancer in the *removed* surgical tissue. It may also be diagnosed as a result of an elevated PSA level leading to a positive prostate biopsy.

Stage B is cancer initially detected as a hard or firm area of the prostate found on digital rectal exam, usually as part of a routine physical exam. If the hard or firm area is small, it is considered a stage B_1 cancer; if larger, a B_2.

Stage C is cancer detected initially by digital rectal exam in which most of the prostate is hard or firm and replaced with cancer. It is also considered a stage C if the cancer has extended up into the seminal vesicle.

Stage D is cancer that has spread *outside* of the prostate. If the spread is just outside the prostate or to lymph nodes near the prostate, it is a stage D_1; if the cancer has spread far from the prostate, say to the lungs or to bones, it is a stage D_2.

Stage A Prostatic Cancer

This is a very unique and unusual form of cancer because its diagnosis is made serendipitously. With this stage of cancer, sometimes known as "occult" prostate cancer, the prostate gland feels entirely normal on rectal examination, there are absolutely no signs or symptoms of cancer and the PSA test may be normal or elevated. Stage A cancer is an "incidental" finding that occurs when a patient has one or more of the various signs and symptoms of voiding difficulty secondary to benign prostatic hyperplasia (see Chapter 4), and the urologist surgically relieves the obstruction to the flow of urine, either by the transurethral route or by one of the "open" surgical approaches (Chapter 6). This incidental stage of prostate cancer is only then diagnosed by the pathologist *after* the surgery, when the removed prostatic tissue (the tissue that has been surgically removed to relieve the symptoms of BPH) is examined microscopically. Such microscopic examination of removed prostatic tissue is always done routinely when surgery is done to relieve the symptoms of BPH, and the report of the pathologist is usually available within two or three days following the prostate surgery. Between 6 and 10 percent of patients who have undergone surgery for what was thought to be BPH, and in whom there was absolutely no reason for any suspicion of cancer, will have been found to have prostate cancer present in the removed surgical specimen. It is this particular group of patients, in whom prostate cancer is a totally unexpected finding, and in whom it would not have been found at all had the patient not undergone surgery for the unrelated problem of BPH, that presents the greatest enigma for urologists. This is because some patients in this group will remain asymptomatic and thrive for many years, while others have a rapid demise in a year or two from a rapidly spreading prostate cancer. Happily, the retrospective studies mentioned earlier have gone far towards clarifying the therapeutic dilemma in which urologists find themselves when this incidental carcinoma is found.

These studies have demonstrated that not all of the incidental carcinomas are the same. In fact, they vary enormously in aggressiveness and behavior; and this variance has been found to be directly related to both the size of the cancer (the tumor bulk) and the microscopic appearance of the cancer (the degree of malignancy, or grade). While all urologists do not agree on the precise and specific details that determine which of these incidental stage A prostatic cancers are less malignant (stage A_1) and which are more malignant (stage A_2), there *is* general agreement that there are *two* kinds of incidental cancer, and although the exact definitions of each of these may vary somewhat from urologist to urologist, certain guidelines are accepted by all. In my opinion, if the incidental cancer found in the removed surgical specimen involves a total tumor bulk that is less than one cubic centimeter and if it is also of low grade when viewed microscopically (grade 1 or 2 on a 1–4 grade scale), then the lesion can be considered an A_1 lesion. If the patient has had a transurethral resection of the prostate for the relief of BPH—and this is by far the most common surgical approach for the treatment of BPH—then a tumor bulk of less than one cubic centimeter can be interpreted to mean that the pathologist has only found microscopic evidence of cancer in three or four chips or pieces of the removed prostate. On the other hand, if the removed specimen is found by the examining pathologist to have more than four or five chips of prostate tissue with cancer in them and / or the microscopic appearance of the tumor is indicative of high-grade malignancy (grade 3 or 4), then the cancer is considered to be an A_2 lesion.

Most urologists agree that true stage A_1 lesions do not need any further therapy and that these are the kinds of prostate cancer that permit great patient longevity and ultimate patient death *with* prostatic cancer but not *from* it. Most urologists also feel the need to verify that the incidental cancer that has been found is indeed a stage A_1 and not merely the "tip of the iceberg" with a more extensive cancer remaining behind after the prostate surgery (recall that the "true" prostate tissue is normally left behind when surgery for BPH is performed). I believe that if a diagnosis of stage A_1 cancer of the prostate is made after an initial operation was done for what was thought to be BPH, it should be followed within a few days or at most a week or two by a repeat operation done transurethrally to see if any cancer has been left behind. An alternative to the repeat transurethral prostate surgery would be multiple biopsies of the prostate under ultrasound control. Still another viable alternative may be to do neither but to follow the patient with PSA levels every 6 months or so and do biopsies only if there is a rising PSA level. If any additional cancer is found, then by definition the patient is no longer considered as having an A_1 cancer but is now upgraded to the A_2 level. Those patients with no remaining cancer following the second transurethral resection or the biopsies remain classified as having A_1 cancers and do not require any specific therapy. However, I feel more comfortable seeing these A_1 patients annually for a digital rectal examination of the prostate and I generally follow them with serial PSA blood tests. In fact, the majority of A_1 prostate cancer patients live out a normal life span and may well not require that anything further be done, of either a diagnostic or a therapeutic nature. However, perhaps a quarter of the patients classified originally as having A_1 do develop additional prostatic cancer over the years, which then puts them into the A_2 category, and this usually requires vigorous therapy.

For that group of patients found to have an A_2 lesion at the time of initial prostatic surgery for what was thought to be BPH, a major therapeutic effort should be undertaken, because these conditions are very different from the A_1 lesions and may be highly malignant. About one-fourth of patients with A_2 lesions will already, at the time of discovery of the cancer, have had it spread to the regional lymph nodes deep in the pelvis; this may possibly mean that the cancer is no longer curable. Therefore, for those patients in whom the surgical operation done for what was thought to be BPH reveals an A_2 lesion, a thorough diagnostic study should be undertaken as soon as possible to search for any evidence of cancer spread beyond the confines of the prostate gland. This study, known as a "metastatic workup," includes bone scans, bone x-rays, chest x-rays, blood tests for prostate specific antigen, and possibly also a blood acid phosphatase. Sometimes a radio-isotope scan of the liver and spleen is done, but this is not usually necessary. If all of these studies suggest that there has been no demonstrable spread of the cancer beyond the confines of the prostate gland, then the patient is considered to be curable pending an additional operation in which the abdomen is opened so that the lymph nodes deep inside the pelvis, which drain the prostate gland, can be removed and examined. These lymph nodes are the nodes within the body to which prostate cancer tends to spread once it has gone beyond the confines of the prostate gland. This is very much analogous to, although obviously much more serious than, the spread of bacteria from a badly inflamed throat to the regional lymph nodes in the neck causing an enlargement of those lymph nodes.

There is no way of establishing with certainty whether the prostate cancer has already spread to one or more of these lymph nodes short of an actual surgical removal of the nodes followed immediately by an examination of them done microscopically by a pathologist. This examination takes about twenty minutes and is done with a "frozen section" technique while the patient is still on the operating table. The frozen section technique is simply a method of freezing and then microscopically examining removed tissue. This method permits a pathologist to render a diagnosis about such tissue in 20–30 minutes whereas the standard (when there is no hurry) technique of preparing and examining removed tissue can take 24 hours.

If microscopic examination of the removed lymph nodes suggests that there is no cancer in any of them, then the pre-

ferred course at this point in time is to remove the entire
prostate gland, performing an operation known as a radical
or total prostatectomy (see Chapter 6). If one or more of the
lymph nodes are found to have cancer in them, then the surgeon's judgment about the potential curability of the cancer
will come into play. Most urologists will back off and not proceed any further if one or more lymph nodes are grossly
involved with tumor; this means that one or more of these
lymph nodes are actually enlarged well beyond their normal
size and the enlargement is due to cancer within the nodes (as
determined by the pathologist). If there is only a microscopic
focus of cancer in one or more of the removed lymph nodes,
some urologists advocate proceeding with the radical removal
of the prostate anyway. Although it is possible that a patient
may well be beyond cure once cancer has entered *any* lymph
nodes, I feel that removal of these lymph nodes with minimal
areas of cancer within them and removal of the entire prostate gland at the same time may well serve to prolong a patient's
life and to improve the quality of his life as well. To be sure,
some centers have recently presented very strong evidence to
suggest that proceeding with a radical prostatectomy and a
bilateral orchiectomy—removal of the testes— in the face of
microscopic *or* gross tumor involvement of one or more lymph
nodes may well dramatically increase the long-term anticipated survival of these patients.

An alternative form of treatment for the patient with stage
A_2 cancer is that of radiation therapy to the prostate and surrounding areas. But the lymph nodes draining the prostate
gland should first be surgically removed and examined, exactly
as noted above, because it is doubtful if radiation therapy will
cure a patient who has lymph node involvement (an alternative method of removing these lymph nodes is via laparos-
copy—see Chapter 9). Since the side effects and complications
of radiation therapy can be significant, this type of treatment
should probably not be done except when there is a reasonable expectation of a cure. It is not at all rare, for example,
for the effects of radiation therapy on the bladder (which,
you will recall, is right next to the prostate) to render the patient
a "urologic cripple" with a resulting permanent need to uri-

nate every ten to thirty minutes, often accompanied by a pronounced urgency. Moreover, about half of the patients receiving radiation therapy become impotent as a result. However, if examination of the lymph nodes is negative, radiation therapy for stage A_2 prostatic cancer is an acceptable form of therapy for the patient who is not, for medical reasons, able to undergo a major operation such as a total removal of the prostate or who otherwise refuses this operation for some reason (see Chapter 6 for additional discussion about radiation therapy). If a patient has required a second transurethral operation on the prostate to make the definitive diagnosis of a stage A_2 cancer, radiation therapy may actually be the best treatment, assuming negative involvement by the lymph nodes, because performing radical or total prostatectomy after two transurethral operations on the prostate is very difficult and is not really a very satisfactory operation. As a general rule, however, I believe that radical surgery offers better long-term results with fewer complications than radiation therapy, although there are unquestionably many excellent physicians who feel that radiation therapy is preferable. Either of these treatment alternatives will offer the best chance of success in the small cancer that is confined within the prostate gland. The option that is best for a given patient will often depend on many factors so that a decision as to which treatment method should be pursued is really best left to the patient and his physician.

Stage B Prostatic Cancer

Perhaps 20 to 30 percent of men with prostatic carcinoma have stage B disease when it is initially diagnosed. It is to identify and diagnose this stage that annual digital rectal examinations of the prostate are recommended. Stage B disease is considered to be curable, and it is divided into B_1 and B_2 lesions. A B_1 lesion is defined as a firm or hard area on the prostate that is less than one to two centimeters in its greatest dimension. A B_2 lesion is one that is greater than two centimeters or that is present on both sides of the prostate gland. On digital rectal examination, a B_1 or B_2 lesion will most classically feel like one or more rock-hard areas on the prostate gland, or, perhaps even more commonly, a firm ridge-like or nodular area that is distinctly different from the feel of the surrounding prostate but is not truly rock-hard. Lesions such as these B lesions are entirely asymptomatic, as are the A lesions, and there is literally nothing to make the patient even remotely aware that he might have cancer in his prostate gland. For this reason, the absolute necessity of including a digital rectal examination of the prostate as part of a periodic physical examination becomes apparent since it is *only* by feeling an abnormality of the prostate gland and pursuing this with biopsies of the abnormal area that there is any chance of making a diagnosis while the condition is still in a curable stage.

After the stage B tumor has been palpated and suspected, skinny-needle aspiration and / or tru-cut biopsy is carried out. Once the prostate cancer has been diagnosed, it is then necessary to stage the cancer in much the same manner as was done for a stage A lesion. This is done to be certain that the cancer is indeed truly a stage B cancer, which, by definition, is confined within the prostate gland. Chest x-rays, bone scans, bone x-rays, and perhaps acid and alkaline phosphatase blood levels are all done; if none of these studies suggest an extension of the cancer outside the prostate gland, the patient is then ready for a staging lymph node removal much as has already been discussed. If none of the removed nodes show any evidence of cancer within them, then the patient is considered to be curable and a total removal of the prostate is carried out. As I have already noted in discussing the stage A cancers, even those patients in whom the cancer has already spread to the lymph nodes of the pelvis may still have a long-term survival and an improved quality of life if they undergo a radical prostatectomy and a bilateral orchiectomy. I recognize that this last statement is not in harmony with prevailing urologic opinion, but the recent work at some major centers strongly supports this aggressive form of therapy. Why the orchiectomy (removal of the testes) as well as the radical prostatectomy? Recall from the earlier definition of the stages of prostate cancer that a stage D cancer is one that has spread outside of the prostate gland. If a patient thought to have an

A, B, or C prostate cancer is found to have cancer in one or more lymph nodes, then by definition that cancer is restaged to a D lesion; if the cancer is *only* in the lymph nodes, it is a D_1 cancer. The preferred treatment for stage D cancers is bilateral orchiectomy (see below and Chapter 6). Undoubtedly, one of the reasons for the remarkable results of the recent past showing long-term survival of prostate cancer patients *with* lymph node involvement following radical prostatectomy has been because bilateral orchiectomy has been carried out during the same operation.

As with stage A prostate cancer, an alternative form of therapy to total prostate removal, after the lymph nodes have been examined and found to be negative for any cancer, would be radiation therapy. I feel, however, that x-ray therapy is clearly a second-choice alternative to total removal of the prostate and that it should be the first-choice treatment only for those patients whose health will not permit a major surgical procedure or for those who refuse it (see discussion of radiation therapy in Chapter 6). For the stage B lesions, and A_2 lesions as well, it is true that radiation therapy has produced very good long-term results in some patients. Many of these long-term cancer survivors, however, are alive *with* the prostate cancer still present, a situation documented by the high percentage of radiation therapy patients who still have positive (for cancer) biopsies of the prostate several months to several years after the radiation therapy has been given. It is because of this, because of the side effects of radiation therapy, and because of my own thirty years of clinical experience in treating patients with prostate cancer that I feel that radical surgery is the best method of treating patients whose cancer is still confined within the prostate.

Stage C Prostatic Cancer

A stage C prostate cancer is more advanced and larger than the A or B stage. On digital rectal examination it is estimated to be a stage C cancer when virtually the entire prostate feels very firm or hard or, alternatively, when the cancer feels as if it has extended up behind the base of the prostate and into the seminal vesicles. About 30 to 40 percent of all prostate cancers are in this stage when first diagnosed. As with stage A and stage B cancers, stage C cancer does not produce any symptoms and the patient is entirely unaware of having this life-threatening condition within his body. It is not uncommon for patients with stage C (or even with any other stage of prostate cancer) to have symptoms of bladder outlet obstruction, but the overwhelming majority of these patients will have coexisting benign prostatic hyperplasia as the cause of these symptoms, since the age group for both of these diseases is virtually the same. Other than some voiding difficulty, which really is not related to prostate cancer in any way, stage C cancer gives no hint of its presence. By definition, a stage C cancer is still confined within the prostate gland and possibly the seminal vesicles as well, and it is therefore still potentially curable. However, it is very common to find at the time of surgical exploration of the lymph nodes done for staging purposes that the cancer in fact has extended beyond the confines of the prostate gland and into the area immediately around the prostate, or into one or more lymph nodes. In either of these situations, the cancer then is considered to be in the stage D category and it may perhaps not be curable. As has already been noted in discussing prostate cancers that were originally thought to be stage A or stage B and were then found to actually be in the lymph nodes (and therefore stage D), the treatment for these patients is variable. Some urologists feel that it is best to proceed with a total removal of the prostate; others feel it best to stop and not remove the prostate because the patient is probably beyond cure.

Many of the patients who are thought to have stage C lesions, based upon the digital rectal examination, will have elevation of their prostate specific antigen levels even though the bone scans and x-rays are negative. In my opinion, an elevated PSA level above 100 ng / ml is pretty strong evidence that a patient in fact has a stage D lesion, but lesser PSA values may also mean that the prostate cancer has spread outside of the prostate gland. Because of this high percentage of patients who are originally thought to be stage C (curable) but who turn out to be stage D (may not be curable), some urologists feel it best just to go ahead with radiation therapy without examining the lymph nodes. I believe that the rationale of these urologists is that 1) the lymph nodes will most likely be positive, so that 2) the patient can't be cured with surgery, and therefore 3) why put the patient through the surgery and 4) go ahead and use radiation therapy because there is nothing else to do. I do not agree with this thinking because I am not at all sure a patient cannot be greatly helped by surgery in terms of longevity and quality of life even if some of his lymph nodes do have cancer in them. I am also convinced that radiation therapy is not beneficial, and may well be harmful because of its side effects, when the cancer has spread to the lymph nodes.

I feel that stage C patients in whom all studies suggest that the cancer is still confined within the prostate should have their lymph nodes examined and, if negative, a radical prostatectomy is best. If there are one or more nodes with microscopic areas of tumor in them, I generally still proceed with radical surgery. Even if there is grossly visible enlargement of lymph nodes with cancer, it may at times still be beneficial to a patient's long-term survival to proceed with radical surgery and bilateral orchiectomy. This decision is often made at the operating table depending on the extent of the visible and gross cancer in the lymph nodes.

In my assessment of patients thought to have a stage C lesion, if the PSA blood test is elevated but all other tests are normal, I still recommend exploration of the nodes and I would handle the situation as just outlined.

Until several years ago, I believed that any patient with prostate cancer in his lymph nodes (even microscopic) was no longer curable. I think that most urologists probably still believe this to be true. However, I now have shifted my thinking because of the very large number of stage D_1 patients who have now been followed for five, ten, and even fifteen years and are alive and seemingly well. All of these patients had prostate cancer in their lymph nodes, but the surgeons did not back off but proceeded with lymph node removal, radical prostatectomy, and bilateral orchiectomy. I still, in my own mind, question whether such patients are truly cured, but I am convinced that the long-term survivals are genuine and that it is far better to proceed with the radical surgery than to back off and let nature take its course.

Stage D Prostatic Cancer

A stage D lesion is one that has spread beyond the confines of the prostate gland. If this spread is by direct growth through the true capsule of the prostate and into the area immediately outside the prostate, or if the spread of the cancer is into the regional lymph nodes of the pelvis, it is a stage D_1 lesion. Stage D prostate cancer typically produces no symptoms at all. If the cancer has spread a great distance from the prostate gland such as to one or more bones or to the lungs or the liver, it is considered to be a stage D_2 lesion. These D_2 lesions may or may not produce any symptoms, although if there has been spread of the cancer to bone there will often be bone pain, which can be very severe; it results from the prostate cancer invading the bone to a degree sufficient to cause bone destruction. It is a truism among urologists, and should hopefully be so among all physicians, that when a man over 50 comes to a physician with pronounced bone pain in the back, the bony pelvis, the hips, or the long bones of the upper legs, the physician should think very rapidly of the possibility of metastatic carcinoma of the prostate. Appropriate bone scans, bone x-rays, and a serum prostatic specific antigen, should be done, as should a careful digital rectal examination of the prostate gland. Probably 30 to 40 percent of all cancers of the prostate are initially diagnosed when they are already stage D and therefore probably not curable. As already noted, however, there are very good data coming from some medical centers suggesting that D_1 lesions with minimal or moderate cancer involvement of the lymph nodes can indeed be treated with an excellent expectation of long-term survival following a radical or total prostatectomy and bilateral orchiectomy. The preponderance of urologic opinion, however, still holds that a patient is probably beyond cure if there is cancer found in the lymph nodes of the pelvis.

The role of radiation therapy in stage D disease is indeed

limited if there is lymph node involvement with cancer. However, when total removal of the prostate gland is done for what was thought to be a stage C lesion, with negative lymph nodes, and the pathologist discovers that the cancer had actually grown through the true capsule of the prostate so that some cancer cells were undoubtedly left in the patient, postoperative radiation therapy to the area where the removed prostate was formerly located might well be indicated.

Since all urologists agree that stage D_2 lesions are certainly incurable and most feel that D_1 lesions may well be incurable, therapy for these advanced forms of prostate cancer are considered to be *palliative* and *not* curative. Certainly surgery and / or radiation therapy is probably not going to cure a patient who has *extensive* spread of cancer beyond the confines of the prostate. And, unfortunately, chemotherapy with any of the presently existing anti-cancer drugs has not been found to be beneficial enough to recommend it as routine treatment. While some specific drugs have achieved temporary relief of symptoms in a small percentage of patients, the use of chemotherapy at this time remains in the experimental or research category. A major question exists, therefore, as to the best treatment for a patient who has an elevated prostate specific antigen level alone (with or without having an elevated acid phosphatase) in the presence of normal bone scans , abdominal CT scans, and normal bone x-rays and who has *not* had any surgery to examine and remove the lymph nodes. Should such surgery be done? I feel that the new prostate specific antigen is accurate enough so that its elevation above 100 ng / ml (and sometimes less)is sufficient proof that the cancer is at least a stage D_1. At this point, the philosophy of the urologist regarding the curability or the incurability of stage D_1 lesions will determine whether to recommend simple palliation to the patient (see below under hormonal therapy) or to aggressively pursue a surgical cure.

If you are wondering about the seeming lack of agreement regarding the treatment options for the different stages of prostate cancer, remember that the seeming confusion is but a reflection of the fact that there is still much that remains unknown about this disease and much that is yet to be learned about it. My own feelings have changed considerably in the very recent past because of convincing data that long-term survivals, virtually the same as the life expectancy without cancer, can be achieved in patients with D_1 cancers by a combination of aggressive surgery and hormonal manipulation (bilateral orchiectomy). Specifically, with a patient having an elevated prostate specific antigen level and *no other* evidence of cancer spread (negative chest x-ray, CT scans, bone scans, and bone x-rays), I do feel that surgical exploration and removal of the lymph nodes *and* a radical prostatectomy is the best treatment. I feel that this offers a patient the best chance at prolonging his life and increasing the quality of his life, even when there is definite cancer already in the lymph nodes. Whether or not to proceed with the radical prostatectomy in the face of definite cancer in the lymph nodes becomes, for me, a judgment call. Certainly, a very extensive amount of cancer outside of the prostate would speak *against* proceeding with the radical prostate removal. Also, since by definition I am speaking of D_1 cancers (spread outside the prostate and into the nearby lymph nodes), I feel that simultaneous hormonal manipulation is best done right at the time of the radical prostatectomy.

My comments here apply to the patient known or suspected of having a D_1 cancer as well as to those patients initially thought to have a stage A or B or even C lesion. If at the time of surgery there is *any* evidence of cancer in a lymph node, then that patient must immediately be reconsidered to have a D_1 lesion. My remarks then become just as applicable to these patients who have been upgraded to a D_1 status as to those patients felt from the beginning to have a D_1 lesion.

I think a word about the upper limits of age for patients having radical prostate surgery is applicable. The standard rule of thumb has always been that a patient over 70 years of age should not have radical prostate surgery, presumably because his life expectancy *without* the cancer is not too different from what it might be *with* the cancer. In general, I tend to agree with the age 70 rule. However, when a patient is in excellent condition and he is a physiological age 65 even though a chronological 75, I think that exceptions should be made.

Certainly, for all stage D_2 lesions, hormonal therapy alone is the treatment of choice. For many patients with D_1 lesions in whom aggressive surgical therapy is not felt to be warranted, either because of the patient's wishes, the urologist's philosophy, or the patient's state of general health, hormonal therapy is also the treatment of choice. The best time to begin this hormonal therapy, however, is unclear, and there is a considerable difference of opinion among urologists on this point. There is even a divergence of opinion about the preferred method of doing the hormonal therapy.

Hormonal Therapy for Stage D Prostate Cancer

Ninety percent of prostate cancers are androgen dependent; this means that the growth of these cancers is enhanced by the influence of the male hormone (androgens). The presence of these androgens, which circulate normally in the male, actually aids and abets the growth and spread of the prostate cancer. The other 10 percent of prostate cancers are not androgen dependent; this means that the growth and rate of spread of these cancers bear no particular relationship to the presence or absence or quantity of male hormones circulating in the body.

For the vast majority (90 percent) of patients with stage D prostate cancer, reduction of the circulating testosterone to near zero levels has been proven to slow down the rate of growth of the cancer and to make the patient feel better although it must be reiterated that this form of treatment is palliative *only* and *not* curative.

There are several ways of markedly reducing the level of male hormones in the body to therapeutic levels. The most obvious is the removal of both testes, called bilateral orchiectomy. Another often-used method is to give estrogen (female hormone) tablets; this will also decrease the circulating male hormone to near zero levels. Unfortunately, the excess estrogen that results from taking estrogen tablets has been shown to have adverse side effects on the heart and major blood vessels and can quite possibly cause cardiovascular complications in more patients than it palliates.

Yet another method to lower the circulating testosterone level has come to light quite recently. Certain hormones act on the male pituitary to initially cause an outpouring of additional testosterone. This might seem paradoxical, but after about a week of this action on the pituitary these hormones cause the testosterone level to drop to near zero, which is about the level achieved when both testes are removed. The reason for this effect is poorly understood, but the action itself is highly reproducible and valid. The hormones that act on the pituitary are known as luteinizing hormone-releasing hormones (LH-RH), and they are given in the form of monthly injections that are administered by a doctor or a nurse. This must be kept up indefinitely, and how faithfully it will actually be done by patients, and whether or not it will be given properly so that the hormone is absorbed and able to act throughout the body, are both questionable. The LH-RH hormones are also very expensive. For these reasons, orchiectomy is without any doubt considered to be the "gold standard" for palliation of prostate cancer, although the injections of LH-RH hormones are probably an acceptable alternative for those patients who refuse orchiectomy.

Another class of drugs used in the treatment of advanced prostate cancer (stage D) are the antiandrogens such as Flutamide and cyproterone acetate. But these really offer nothing beyond what has been mentioned above, although some studies have shown a slightly increased survival when Flutamide is given along with the LH-RH agonist. Ketaconazole is an antifungal drug that has also been found to act as an antiandrogen but all of these drugs have their drawbacks. These drawbacks are twofold: first, drugs given by mouth are, at times, absorbed through the stomach and into the bloodstream in a very capricious manner, so that the circulating blood level of the drug is not necessarily at therapeutic levels all the time. Second, the problem of compliance is always a problem since many patients actually do not take their medicine when they are feeling well or when they simply forget to take it. For these reasons, removal of the testes must remain, for the patient who will agree to it, as the standard against which these drugs must be compared.

Another major question about the palliative hormonal treatment for stage D cancer about which there is a great deal of controversy concerns the optimum time to begin such therapy. The early landmark studies of the late 1930s and 1940s conclusively demonstrated that androgen deprivation (orchiectomy) prolonged the life of patients with stage D prostate cancer and also improved the quality of life remaining to the patient. Various researchers have attempted to determine whether it made any significant difference in the patient's life expectancy or in his quality of life if the androgen deprivation was initiated at the time that stage D cancer was diagnosed, or if the therapy was held in abeyance until the patient developed symptoms of the cancer spread. Most commonly the symptoms of stage D prostate cancer were pain that occurred when the cancer spread to bone. A very extensive study done on a cooperative basis by many hospitals of the Veterans Administration suggested that the total life expectancy from the time that stage D disease was diagnosed until death was about the same whether the treatment was begun at the time of diagnosis or at the time that the metastatic disease produced symptoms. This study showed that if treatment began at the time of diagnosis there was a longer symptom-free interval until the patient developed pain in the bones; but then the interval from the onset of pain until death was shorter than if the androgen deprivation treatment was delayed until the painful symptoms of bone metastases developed. Urologists at present are fairly divided as to whether it is best to recommend the orchiectomy, or some alternative procedure such as LH-RH hormones or even estrogen (rarely), at the time that the stage D disease is diagnosed or to wait until the patient develops the symptoms of bone pain. I believed formerly that it was preferable to delay the treatment until symptoms developed because in that manner the best weapon to alleviate the pain and suffering of metastatic disease was saved until it was actually needed. More recently, I have changed my mind because new data from large numbers of patients suggests strongly that patients may live significantly longer, and with a better quality of life, if the hormonal therapy is begun at the time that the patient's stage D cancer is first diagnosed.

Survival Statistics

As we have seen, cancer of the prostate can almost be considered to be many different diseases because the activity of the cancer varies enormously from patient to patient. However, it does appear quite clear that the larger the size of the cancer and the higher its microscopic grade at the time of diagnosis, the poorer the outlook for survival. For those cancers that are extremely small and of low microscopic grade (stage A_1), the survival will probably be about the same as it would be for an individual without prostate cancer. These very small, sometimes microscopic, foci of prostate cancer represent the kind of cancer that patients die *with* and not *from,* and it is this kind of cancer (A_1) that I am referring to when I say that up to 30 percent of men over age 50 have cancer of the prostate. The other kind of prostate cancer that is not possible to detect on digital rectal examination is the stage A_2 lesion. By definition, the A_2 lesion is more extensive and usually of a higher grade than the A_1 lesion. The A_2 lesion should not be thought of as a condition of low malignancy, however, and probably up to 25 percent of these tumors have already spread to regional lymph nodes at the time of original diagnosis.

Once there is definite evidence that the tumor has spread to lymph nodes it is much less likely that a cure can be brought about. The five-year survival rate has traditionally been reported to be no better than 50 percent, with a ten-year survival of around 30 percent in those patients with cancer already in their lymph nodes. I think it is important for the reader to realize that all of the "survival" figures given in this section are the traditional ones that have been reported over the years, and they do *not* reflect the extraordinary improvement in survival data from the very aggressive surgical approach discussed in this chapter (see Chapter 9 for this newer survival data). I firmly believe that once this very new data becomes generally accepted, more urologists will alter their philosophies of treatment and the traditional survival data will reflect this.

For those lesions that are thought to be B_1 or B_2 based on digital rectal examination, about 15 percent of the B_1 patients and 25 or 30 percent of the B_2 patients will turn out to have lymph node involvement with cancer at the time of surgical exploration, a fact that automatically changes the stage to a D_1. If all of the lymph nodes are "clean" and no cancer is found in them, however, better than an 80 percent ten-year survival can be anticipated. If any lymph nodes are found to have cancer in them, the survival statistics for the stages B_1 and B_2 cancers are about the same as for the stage A_2 lesions.

When the cancer is initially felt to be a stage C, surgical exploration and examination of the lymph nodes will show cancer already in these nodes about half of the time. As a general rule, once lymph node involvement with cancer has occurred the standard patient survival statistics are pretty much the same regardless of the stage of the cancer that was initially thought to exist. They are all stage D by definition, once there is cancer in the lymph nodes. Most will be considered for palliation as opposed to an attempt at surgical cure. Not all stage D cancers are the same, however, and the higher the microscopic grade the poorer the survival statistics. If bony metastases are present at the time of initial diagnosis of any stage of prostate cancer, the survival for five years is under 50 percent and probably much nearer to 30 percent.

The reader will discern from some of these survival statistics that a cancer initially thought to be stage A or stage B is not necessarily so at the time of surgical examination of the lymph nodes and that, of course,. is the reason that a meticulous examination of the lymph nodes is necessary prior to proceeding with a radical, total removal of the prostate. The initial staging of a tumor is based upon the digital rectal examination, the prostate specific antigen blood level (only if very high), and also on bone scans, CT scans, bone x-rays, and chest x-rays. Additionally, the PSA blood level, if it is very high, may be of significance in indicating whether or not there has been any spread of the cancer. The results of all of these studies taken together give what is referred to as a clinical staging of the tumor. But probably a third of the time, or even more, surgical exploration leads to an upgrading of the tumor stage as a result of finding cancer in the lymph nodes. This gives the urologist a pathologic stage, which is really the most important one and the one upon which treatment is usually based.

In this chapter the survival data presented will undoubtedly lead many readers to the obvious question: Why shouldn't the five-year survival rate be 100 percent when the lymph nodes show *no* evidence of tumor involvement and all other tests are similarly negative for the presence of prostate cancer? This is, of course, a central question to survival data for any cancer, but the less than 100 percent survival is because of the unfortunate fact that there has indeed been spread of the cancer outside of the confines of the prostate gland, but the spread has been a microscopic one and not detectable. For example, when the lymph nodes are removed so that the pathologist can examine them to determine the presence or absence of cancer in these lymph nodes, only a random sampling of nodes are removed from those areas which represent the highest likelihood, anatomically speaking, of cancer spread. It is certainly possible that some lymph nodes not removed do indeed have microscopic foci of cancer. The reason that all lymph nodes are not removed at this staging operation is because when this is done, and radiation therapy to the pelvis is subsequently required, a massive and very unpleasant swelling of the lower extremities, the penis, and the scrotum will often result. In fact, the vast majority of prostate cancers that do spread to lymph nodes will do so in a highly predictable pattern, so it is the lymph nodes to which the spread is predicted that are removed and sampled. Another reason for the less than 100 percent cure rate in patients with negative nodes is that spread of the cancer to bone may have already occurred at the time of the lymph node sampling and removal, but the changes in the bone were too early to be detected on bone scans or bone x-rays.

In summary, cure of the patient with prostate cancer ideally depends upon the total removal of the prostate gland before any spread of the cancer outside of the gland has occurred. The smaller the cancer is initially, the greater the likelihood of accomplishing this; conversely, the larger the tumor present initially, the greater the likelihood of its having already spread outside of the prostate, possibly rendering it beyond cure. Additional factors in survival are the microscopic appearance of the tumor which is graded on a 1–4 scale; the higher the grade the more malignant the tumor. Finally, the intangible and immeasurable factor of the biologic potential of *any* cancer and the patient's resistance to that cancer are factors to be considered but are not factors that can be measured.

6

Surgical Procedures and Radiation Therapy

QUESTION: What did the fortieth president of the United States have in common with almost 400,000 other American men?

ANSWER: In 1987, all of these individuals had surgery to relieve the symptoms of benign prostatic hyperplasia (BPH); and the vast majority of these operations (including that of the president) were done using the transurethral approach.

In this chapter I am going to discuss in some detail exactly how prostate surgery is performed. This discussion will include, in addition to the most frequently used transurethral approach, the other surgical approaches for BPH. I will also discuss those operations that are done in an effort to cure prostate cancer (radical prostatectomy). I recognize that not all readers will want to read this chapter since it might be more technical than some of you would like, and because it isn't always pleasant to read about surgical procedures that may be carried out on oneself. Nevertheless, for those interested in knowing precisely what will be done to them when they have prostate surgery, I hope that this chapter will provide the answers.

I also feel it is appropriate in this chapter to make some

general statements about radiation therapy for cancer of the prostate, how it is done, and its short-term and long-term side effects. Finally, I think it appropriate to go into some detail about the surgery done for removal of the testes (bilateral orchiectomy) since this procedure is done, or at least recommended, quite frequently for the treatment of prostate cancer that has already spread outside the limits of the prostate gland.

Surgery for Benign
Prostatic Hyperplasia (BPH)

There are four surgical approaches used in the treatment of BPH. Selection of the operation best suited to the individual patient is fundamental to a successful result (Fig. 6–1).

The transurethral approach is done entirely through the penis, while the suprapubic and retropubic approaches require abdominal incisions and so are known as "open" operations. All are in common usage. The perineal approach, also an open operation, is infrequently used. Each of these four approaches has its advantages and disadvantages. Sometimes, circumstances permit only one acceptable approach to the operation; at other times two or more options are available. Not infrequently, a surgeon may feel more comfortable with one approach than with another, representing perhaps the emphasis of his training and also his own experience with the different approaches since completing his training. You should feel quite free to discuss the proposed surgical approach with your urologist; you should also feel completely satisfied with the explanation that he gives you. It is your body and it is your money, and I, for one, feel that the better informed a patient is about a surgical procedure the more rapid his recovery may be and the better the result that he will obtain. Not all patients care to know much about the details of their operation, and that is, of course, perfectly all right.

The transurethral approach is unquestionably the one most commonly used, and it also is by far the least disturbing and least painful for the patient. However, this approach requires

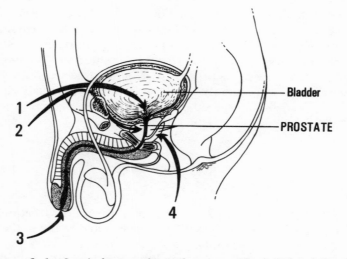

Figure 6–1   *Surgical approaches to the prostate gland. This is a lateral view of a man, through the midportion of his body, and shows the four most frequently used approaches for the surgical treatment of BPH: 1) the suprapubic approach; 2) the retropubic approach; 3) the transurethral approach, called a TURP and by far the most commonly used approach; and 4) the perineal approach, very infrequently used.*

infinitely more surgical skill than any of the open surgical procedures; and most urologists consider that the transurethral approach, because of its inherent difficulty which is magnified by a very large prostate, should not be used if the estimated size of the prostate tissue (the BPH) to be removed is much over about 50 grams. As it happens, however, only about 10 percent of all patients requiring surgery for BPH have more than 50 grams of BPH tissue to be removed.

One of the open surgical approaches may be preferred occasionally, even for relatively small prostate glands, if there are other procedures that need to be done at the same time such as the removal of one or more large stones from the bladder or the excision of any bladder diverticula that are present. Another indication for an open procedure through the abdomen is for those patients with a severe limitation of hip movement that precludes the use of the lithotomy position necessary for transurethral surgery. The lithotomy position is one in which the patient is flat on his back with the legs spread widely apart and elevated by placing leg supports behind the knees. These instances notwithstanding, open surgical procedures are done very infrequently. At my own institution, more than 97 percent of the 250 surgeries carried out each year for BPH are done via the transurethral route.

The remainder of this chapter, dealing with specific details of the different surgical approaches to benign prostatic hyperplasia will be easier to understand if you keep in mind a few anatomic facts that were pointed out in Chapter 1. Each of the surgical approaches to BPH is based on the same principle: all of the tissue that is *within* the surgical capsule must be removed, leaving behind the true prostate tissue and the true capsule of the prostate. In doing this it should be understood that the prostatic urethra itself will be removed and will be replaced naturally by a new lining that will grow down from the bladder. Remembering the analogy of the apple with the core removed in which the hole through the apple represents the prostatic urethra, you will recall that it is just under the lining of the prostatic urethra that the BPH begins to grow. If it grows in an inward direction it will obstruct the channel of the prostatic urethra. It may, and usually does, also grow in an outward direction giving an enlarged feel to the prostate on digital rectal examination. As the BPH grows in an outward direction it compresses the true prostate tissue between itself and the true capsule of the prostate. Between the expanding growth of BPH and the true prostate tissue there is a plane which is called the surgical capsule. As used here, a "plane" refers merely to the point at which two separate tissues, the BPH and the true prostate, touch one another. The surgical "capsule" is not a capsule at all but simply the name given to the interface between the BPH tissue and the true prostate tissue. It may be visualized as the relationship between a piece of scotch tape and a piece of cloth on which the tape is resting. The surgical capsule would be the interface of the sticky side of the tape and the cloth. The surgical treatment of BPH involves removing all of the tissue that is within (inside of) the surgical capsule leaving behind the true prostate tissue and the true capsule. The tissue that is being removed is only the BPH itself, and it includes the lining of the prostatic urethra (Fig. 6–2). The only differences between the four principal surgical procedures for BPH are in the approach to the BPH tissue itself, but all of the procedures effectively do the same thing.

Anesthesia in Prostate Surgery

Spinal anesthesia, an injection into the spine which blocks pain but leaves the patient awake, is the preferred anesthesia since it ideally combines total absence of pain and complete relaxation of the patient with virtually no postoperative lung problems. It is often difficult to achieve all of these benefits with a general anesthesia, but for the patient who has abnormally low blood pressure and/or certain types of heart problems, general anesthesia may be best since spinal anesthesia may cause acute and sudden lowering of the blood pressure which could present a problem for the patient with existing heart disease. Spinal anesthesia is also often avoided in patients who have had back surgery or spinal cord injuries.

Transurethral Prostate Surgery

The modern era of transurethral prostate surgery (also known as transurethral resection of the prostate, or TURP) goes back to the 1950s. In the intervening years the technique and the instrumentation has been polished and refined so that the operation today may really be said to be as successful and as excellent as any major surgical procedure in terms of low death rate, few complications, and excellent surgical results. The operation is done through the urethra with an instrument that is similar to a cystoscope. When the instrument is positioned within the prostatic urethra, obstructing BPH tissue is cut away, beginning in the center of the prostatic urethra and working towards the periphery of the prostate gland until the surgical capsule is reached. At this point all of the

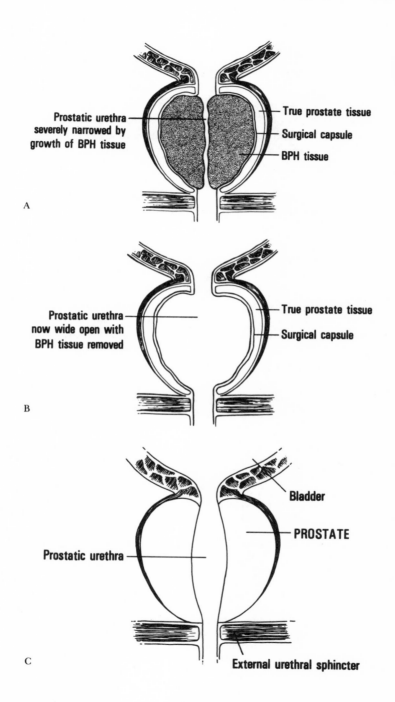

A

Prostatic urethra severely narrowed by growth of BPH tissue

True prostate tissue

Surgical capsule

BPH tissue

B

Prostatic urethra now wide open with BPH tissue removed

True prostate tissue

Surgical capsule

C

Prostatic urethra

Bladder

PROSTATE

External urethral sphincter

BPH should be removed leaving behind only the true prostate tissue.

The TURP is the operation of choice for small and moderate growths of BPH, perhaps up to 50 grams. It is also the indicated operation for patients known to have cancer of the prostate who also have symptoms of bladder outlet obstruction—either due to the cancer or to BPH—but who are not considered suitable patients for total (radical) prostatectomy for some reason. Transurethral prostatic resection is technically difficult to do in patients with massive BPH (over 100 grams), and the upper size limit of BPH that a given urologist will undertake to operate upon will vary according to his skill and experience.

The principal advantages of the transurethral approach are: 1) The patient is usually hospitalized for a much shorter time postoperatively (by several days) than when open surgery is done; and 2) the patient will have far less pain and discomfort and will be eating, walking around, and "feeling good" within twenty-four hours of surgery. The disadvantages of the transurethral approach are: 1) The procedure is technically much more difficult than any of the open procedures, and highly specialized surgical equipment is required; and 2) the risks of considerable loss of blood and of postsurgical urinary incontinence are very real, as are the risks of postoperative bladder neck contracture and urethral stricture

Figure 6–2   THE PROSTATE GLAND BEFORE AND AFTER SURGERY TO RELIEVE BENIGN PROSTATIC HYPERPLASIA.

A. An extensive growth of benign prostatic hyperplasia tissue stretching the true prostate tissue out towards the periphery of the prostate gland and severely encroaching upon the prostatic urethra.

B. The prostate gland following surgery. Note that all of the benign prostatic hyperplasia tissue has been removed, leaving a large prostatic urethra through which urine flows.

C. Within several weeks following surgery the true prostate gland contracts so that the prostatic urethra once again has a configuration such as it did before the BPH started to grow. The compressed true prostate tissue is able to resume its normal configuration, filling the vacancy left by the removal of the BPH tissue.

(see Chapter 8). Even though the surgical instrument used to remove the prostate is inserted through the penis, there is virtually no risk of penile trauma, because the instrument is being placed into a channel (the urethra) that can accommodate it and because no surgery is being done to the penis itself. All of the surgery is being done on the prostate gland and is being done from within the prostate gland. Sexual dysfunctions resulting from the placement of the instrument in the penis are virtually unknown. It should be pointed out that all of the risks and complications noted above are also applicable, to a greater or lesser degree, to the open surgical procedures. Overall, the transurethral approach is the procedure of choice for the skilled urologist competent in all of the surgical approaches. A huge growth of BPH (over 100 grams) would be the principal indication for the choice of an open operation.

There are two types of surgical instrument used in transurethral surgery. Both are referred to as resectoscopes. The instrument that is by far the most widely used employs an electric cutting current to trim away the obstructing prostatic tissue. The other instrument uses a tubular knife blade to cut away the prostatic tissue. The latter instrument was developed and popularized at the Mayo Clinic where it is still used, and it is also used by many of the urologists in this country who trained at the Mayo Clinic.

When either type of resectoscope has been introduced through the urethra and into the bladder, it is possible to note the type and extent of prostatic enlargement that is present. This enlargement will consist of either middle-lobe enlargement, enlargement of the two lateral lobes, or enlargement of all three lobes. The principle of the transurethral approach to prostatic surgery, regardless of the type of resectoscope that is used, is to trim away the obstructing prostatic tissue starting from the inside of the prostatic urethra and working towards the outside of the prostate gland (Fig. 6–3). Imagine putting an instrument inside a very narrow and obstructed core of an apple and then, working from the inside of the core in an outwards direction towards the skin of the apple, trimming away the pulp of the apple until the core is enlarged

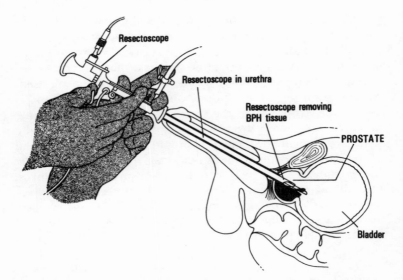

Figure 6–3   *A transurethral resection of the prostate (TURP), showing the surgical instrument (the resectoscope) in the urethra and in the bladder as the surgeon removes pieces of tissue from the prostate gland.*

to the point that there is no tissue/pulp obstructing the channel. Sometimes, this may involve trimming away the obstructing BPH growth until just a very thin rim of tissue may remain just under the true capsule of the prostate. At other times, trimming away the obstructing new growth of prostate (the BPH) may only require the removal of a few pieces of BPH tissue. This is often the case when the obstruction to the flow of urine is caused by middle lobe enlargement alone. Although enlargements of this middle lobe are probably the most common cause of prostatic obstruction, and can produce the most severe symptoms of obstruction, it is interesting that in terms of actual size or amount of obstructing tissue the middle lobe enlargements are usually quite small and often less than 10 or 20 grams in weight. Middle lobe enlargement cannot be detected on digital rectal examination of the prostate gland. Lateral lobe prostatic enlargement, on the other hand, can be very large and extensive in terms of the amount and weight of tissue that needs to be removed in order to relieve the obstruction. It is these massive lateral lobe enlargements that can yield 80 or 100 grams or more of BPH tissue to be removed.

During the course of the actual surgical procedure, which takes perhaps an hour or an hour and a half, many blood vessels—both arteries and veins—are cut across; so bleeding can be considerable. This is the reason that an irrigation system is required, which ensures a continuous supply of fluid flowing through the resectoscope and into the bladder, keeping the surgical field clear of blood while the urologist is trimming away the obstructing BPH tissue. During this continuous irrigation the bladder fills every 20 to 30 seconds, so it becomes necessary to periodically stop the continuous flow, empty the irrigating fluid from the bladder through the resectoscope, and start again. Some urologists prefer to use a type of resectoscope that permits continuous drainage of the irrigating fluid, thereby obviating the need to periodically stop in order to empty the bladder. The pieces of prostate tissue (the BPH) that have been removed up to that point leave the bladder through the resectoscope along with the irrigating fluid. Since it is not possible to clamp and tie off the blood vessels that are cut during the course of surgery, as is done with open operative procedures, these blood vessels must be fulgurated or "cooked" with a coagulating electrical current that both types of resectoscope are able to apply directly to the bleeding blood vessels. The skill of the urologist is of the utmost importance in the outcome of a transurethral prostatic operation in terms of removing all of the obstructing BPH tissue without injuring or destroying normal prostate tissue, being able to control by fulguration the many blood vessels that invariably bleed during surgery, not injuring any of the anatomic areas that control urinary continence, and not damaging the normal bladder neck which can lead to a bladder neck contracture (see Chapter 8).

Following removal of all of the obstructing prostatic tissue, a Foley catheter is placed into the patient's bladder and the balloon is inflated to keep the catheter in place for several days while the very small blood vessels within the prostatic urethra that cannot be coagulated seal themselves off and stop bleeding (Fig. 6–4). The catheter also allows a continuous irrigation of the bladder for a day or so after surgery, in order to minimize clot formation that would act as a foreign body within the bladder and cause painful bladder spasms. Clots would also act to impede the drainage of urine to the outside. For the first couple of days after surgery, the urine drainage through the catheter tends to be bloody, but by the time the catheter is removed on the second or third day following surgery, the urine is usually visibly clear. Microscopic blood will normally persist in the urine for a number of weeks following surgery until the prostatic urethra is entirely healed.

Although the results of this type of surgery are usually excellent, you must remember that when surgery by any approach for the relief of BPH is done, the true prostate tissue is left behind and so also is the cause (which is poorly understood) of the original growth of BPH tissue. Therefore, it must be anticipated that a certain number of individuals will have a regrowth of their BPH tissue, necessitating another operation. Obviously, the younger a man is when he has his prostate surgery, the greater the likelihood of a regrowth

Figure 6–4   *Immediately after the TURP, a Foley catheter is placed through the urethra and into the bladder. This figure shows the catheter in place following a TURP.*

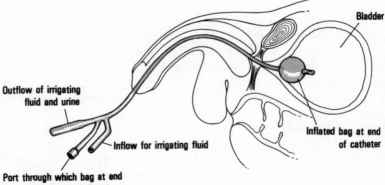

Bladder

Outflow of irrigating
fluid and urine

Inflow for irrigating fluid

Inflated bag at end
of catheter

Port through which bag at end
of catheter is inflated

because he will presumably live for many years after the initial operation. Considering all patients who have prostate surgery for BPH, between 10 and 15 percent will ultimately need another operation. But it must be remembered that this is an age-related phenomenon. An 80-year-old man having his first TUR (transurethral resection) of the prostate is highly unlikely to ever need another one, whereas a 45-year-old man will very likely need another one if he lives long enough.

The Suprapubic Approach

The suprapubic approach (the word "pubic" refers to the pubic bone) to the prostate (suprapubic prostatectomy) is through the lower abdomen, making an opening into the bladder. The prostate is reached with a hand inside the bladder, with the index finger advancing through the bladder neck and down into the prostatic urethra. There are two very similar operations: the "blind" suprapubic approach, and the visual or "open" one.

The "blind" approach, so-called because the entire operation is done by "feel" alone and not under direct vision, was developed in 1896 by Peter Freyer. In 1909 Thompson Walker originated the visual or "open" suprapubic prostatectomy which allowed the operating surgeon to see the surgical field directly and to control bleeding by placing stitches into the bladder neck. The two procedures, however, are really very similar.

Blind Suprapubic Prostatectomy. The principal advantage of this type of operation is that it requires only a minimum of surgical expertise and a minimum of special equipment. It can also be done with something less than excellent abdominal relaxation and exposure of the surgical field; therefore minimal anesthesia expertise is required. The primary disadvantage of this technique is the difficulty in controlling bleeding since the actual bleeding vessels are never visualized. In this day and age of surgical excellence, however, there really are no specific indications for this type of operation except perhaps if the patient is being cared for in an area where there is an absence of surgical assistance and a paucity of specialized urologic instruments. This procedure must *not* be done when a patient is known to have cancer of the prostate because it is frequently not possible to separate and remove the BPH tissue from the underlying true prostate because of the strong possibility that the cancer has spread from the true prostate (where it arose) directly into the BPH tissue (Fig. 6–5). Attempts to remove the obstructing BPH tissue may well result in tearing and ripping the prostate gland right through its true capsule since the usual cleavage plane of the surgical capsule is no longer present because of the cancer. For this same reason, *none* of the open surgical approaches should be used for BPH if cancer is known to be present.

Figure 6–5   *A prostate gland with both benign prostatic hyperplasia and cancer. Note that the cancer tends to grow in an inward direction from the periphery where it arose. In growing in this inward manner, it grows right through the plane of the surgical capsule, thereby making it extremely difficult or even impossible to enucleate or "shell out" the BPH tissue via either the suprapubic, retropubic, or perineal approaches. For this reason, a patient known to have prostate cancer should only have the transurethral approach to the prostate used for the purpose of relieving obstruction to the flow of urine.*

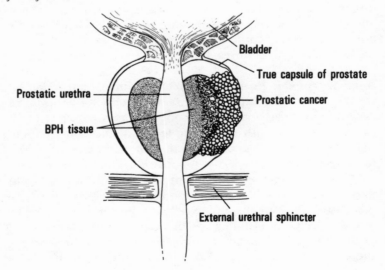

Bladder

True capsule of prostate

Prostatic urethra

Prostatic cancer

BPH tissue

External urethral sphincter

With the patient lying on his back on the operating table, an incision from the navel to the pubic bone is made and extended down through the layers of the abdominal wall until the bladder, which has been distended with water put in through a Foley catheter, is exposed. The bladder is opened and the index finger is placed through the bladder neck and down into the prostatic urethra. Then, that index finger breaks through the urethra in an upwards direction at the level of the far end of the prostate, and the removal of the BPH begins (Fig. 6–6). Recall that in this blind suprapubic approach, as in all of the surgical approaches to BPH, the principle of the surgery is to remove *all* of the tissue that is within the surgical capsule. When the index finger has broken through the prostate urethral lining and the BPH, it will stop at the plane between the BPH and the true prostate tissue (the surgical capsule) because the BPH splits easily before the upward pushing motion of the index finger while the true prostate is

Figure 6–6   *The blind suprapubic surgical approach to the prostate gland in which the finger is inserted into the bladder and then into the prostatic urethra before starting removal of the BPH tissue.*

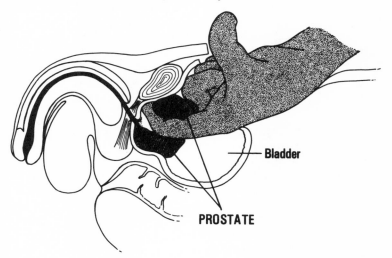

Bladder

PROSTATE

more resistant and does not easily yield. Once the index finger has found the plane between the BPH and the true prostate tissue, the surgeon sweeps the finger around in that plane, embracing an arc of 180° first on one side and then on the other until all of the BPH tissue is separated from the underlying true prostate.

With this operative approach it is not possible for the surgeon to visualize the bladder neck very well; and it certainly is not possible to visualize any part of the interior of the true prostate once the obstructing tissue has been removed. It is therefore not possible to identify any bleeding vessels. Control of bleeding, which can be profuse, is usually done by placing a large gauze pack into the inside of the true prostate gland where it is left for several minutes. This will usually stop the bleeding or reduce it to a minimum. The bladder is then closed with stitches and a large catheter-like tube is brought out of the bladder directly through the lower part of the abdomen, while a smaller Foley catheter is placed into the bladder through the urethra. In this manner, with two catheters to drain the blood and the urine, the likelihood of clot formation plugging both catheters is minimized.

I generally prefer to remove the bladder tube that is coming through the abdominal wall once the drainage from both catheters is relatively free of blood. With the urethral catheter still in place, the opening into the bladder where the removed catheter had been closes spontaneously in a day or two, after which the urethral catheter can be removed. It is generally seven to ten days before the urine is quite clear of blood, both catheters are removed, and the patient is able to go home.

Visual or Open Suprapubic Prostatectomy. The same reasons for doing a blind suprapubic operation apply to the visual procedure; and the reasons for *not* doing the blind operation apply as well. When the visual operation is done, the incision into the bladder is made much closer to the bladder neck so that it is actually possible for the surgeon to see the bladder neck and to control bleeding after the obstructing prostate tissue has been removed. Further, with the visual operation, it is also possible to do a neater and cleaner repair of the denuded bladder neck in the area from which the obstructing prostate tissue was removed. In all other ways, however, the operation is really basically similar to the blind operation. In practice, the vast majority of operations that are now done using the suprapubic approach are done in a manner that permits the surgeon to see the bladder neck and to accomplish reasonably good control of bleeding. The postoperative course is the same for the open as for the blind approach.

The Retropubic Approach

The retropubic approach (retropubic prostatectomy) is the most recently developed of the four presently used approaches for the surgical treatment of BPH. Although it was first utilized in 1909 it was not established on a sound and firm basis until 1945 when the English surgeon Terrence Millen popularized the procedure. This approach, as with the suprapubic approach, is primarily indicated when a massive amount of obstructing prostate tissue is present, an amount that is felt to be too large for the transurethral operation. It is also indicated, as is the suprapubic approach, for those patients whose inability to flex the hips precludes the lithotomy position that is necessary for the transurethral approach. However, as with the suprapubic approach and for the same reason, the retropubic approach should not be used in the presence of cancer of the prostate.

The advantages of the retropubic approach are that it permits very excellent exposure of the prostate gland and of the bladder neck, and thereby greatly facilitates accurate control of bleeding after the obstructing tissue has been removed. The bladder itself is not opened with this approach, and there is no need for a catheter coming through the bladder wall following surgery as is necessary with the suprapubic approach. The disadvantages of the retropubic approach are primarily that very specialized surgical instruments are needed and the exposure of the prostate gland can be extremely difficult in obese men or in those with a particularly narrow or deep bony pelvis.

The operation is usually performed with the patient on

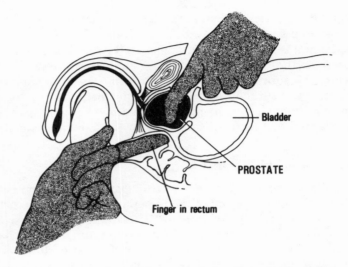

Figure 6–7   *The retropubic approach to the removal of BPH tissue in which the surgeon's finger does not enter the bladder but goes directly through the true capsule of the prostate in order to remove the BPH tissue. The finger in the rectum elevates the prostate and facilitates the surgery.*

his back. The same up-and-down incision is made in the lower abdomen as is made when using the suprapubic approach. The incision is carried through the layers of muscle in the abdomen; then the area *under* the pubic bone is cleaned so that the entire surface of the prostate gland is exposed. Because the surgical exposure is primarily behind and under the pubic bone the operation is known as a *retropubic* prostatectomy. Once the area under the pubic bone and directly over the prostate itself has been visualized, an incision is made in the true capsule of the prostate just below the bladder neck. The incision is deepened through the true prostate tissue and to the plane marking the junction of the true prostate tissue from the growth of BPH tissue (Fig. 6–7). This plane is known as the surgical capsule that has been described before, and when it is reached it is readily recognized. The enucleation or "shelling out" of the BPH tissue is then done all the way around the circumference of the prostate gland, the tissue inside this plane being removed with the surgeon's finger and a long-curved scissors.

The reader should note that this is very similar to the suprapubic operation except that with the latter the enuclea-tion or "shelling out" of the BPH tissue begins in the channel of the prostatic urethra and moves in an outward direction, whereas the retropubic operation begins at the outside of the prostate gland and moves in an inward direction. With both operations the end result is the same. In both operations all of the BPH growth is removed along with the lining of the prostatic urethra, since it is the inner lining of the BPH growth. Bleeding in the retropubic operation is controlled by placing stitches in the bleeding areas which are easy to visualize; therefore the postoperative complication of bleeding is less common than with the suprapubic approach. The bladder neck is trimmed and "neatened," a catheter is advanced through the urethra and into the bladder and left there for a few days, and the incisions in the prostatic capsule and in the abdomi-nal wall are closed.

Perineal Prostatectomy

The oldest, by far, of the four types of surgical exposure for the treatment of BPH is that through the perineum, the area between the scrotum and the anus. This very early oper-ation developed from the ancient "cutting for the stone" or going through the perineal area and into the bladder for the purpose of removing bladder stones. In fact, this operation for stones actually dates from well before the time of Christ. In 1903 the present operation using the perineal approach for relief of BPH was devised by Dr. Hugh Young (Fig. 6–8).

This surgical approach really has very few advantages over the other approaches; in fact, it probably produces a higher incidence of erectile dysfunction (impotence) postoperatively than any of the other approaches (because the nerves that control erections are exposed to possible damage when this surgical approach is used). Since the perineal approach, because of these factors, is so rarely used for the treatment of BPH, I won't describe or discuss it.

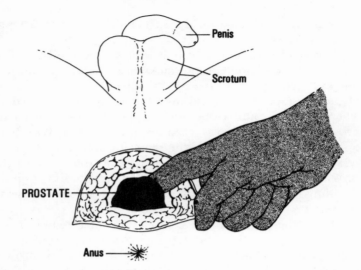

Figure 6–8   *The perineal approach to the removal of BPH tissue in which the incision is made in the area between the patient's anus and scrotum and the prostate gland is approached from below.*

Surgery for Cancer of the Prostate

The preferred treatment, in my estimation, for cancer of the prostate, when the patient's disease is at a stage where a long-term survival or a cure can be anticipated, is the radical or total removal of the prostate gland. This operation is fundamentally and completely different from any and all of those operations already described for the treatment of BPH because the *entire* prostate gland is removed (Fig. 6–9). When the entire prostate is removed in an attempt to cure prostatic cancer, the bladder is brought down into the pelvis and the bladder neck is stitched to the stump of the urethra at the point where the prostate gland was detached from it. In this manner, the gap where the removed prostate had been is bridged and the continuity of the lower urinary tract is reestablished. Obviously,

Retropubic approach

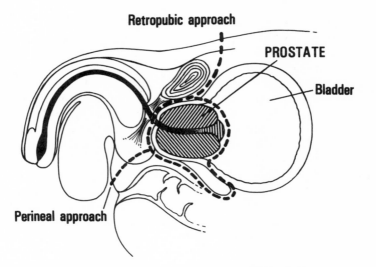

PROSTATE

Bladder

Perineal approach

Figure 6–9   *The principle of radical or total prostatectomy (removal of the prostate) for the treatment of prostate cancer. The dotted lines indicate that the approach can be retropubic or perineal. The dotted lines also indicate that the entire prostate gland and the seminal vesicles (included within the dotted lines) are removed in this type of operation.*

a radical or total prostatectomy is completely unrelated to the four operative procedures for the relief of BPH that we have just discussed. In these four operations the term "prostatectomy" is commonly used, but it is a misnomer since the procedure that is actually done for BPH is a removal of *only* that portion of the prostate gland that is obstructing the flow of urine (the BPH), leaving behind the true prostate tissue and the true capsule of the prostate.

There are two distinct and different surgical procedures that are used when a radical or total prostatectomy is done. The first, and the one which I much prefer, is the retropubic approach. This operation is known as a *radical* or *total retropubic prostatectomy.* It is very different from the operation done for BPH that is known as a "conservative" or "simple" retropubic prostatectomy; but it does use the same surgical approach to the prostate—from behind and under the pubic bone—as the retropubic procedure for BPH. The second surgical procedure for prostate cancer is known as a *radical perineal prostatectomy*. It uses the same approach (through the perineum) as the simple or conservative perineal prostatectomy that is very infrequently used in the treatment of BPH.

The primary advantage of the retropubic approach to a radical prostatectomy is that it permits the removal and examination of the lymph nodes of the pelvis, to which prostate cancer tends to spread. The nodes are known as the obturator, the external, and the internal iliac lymph nodes, and it is these nodes that are removed and examined microscopically as part of the staging procedure to see if a prostate cancer is confined within the prostate gland. The lymph nodes are examined and the results reported within about twenty minutes, using an examining technique known as a "frozen" section. As we have seen, there is no concensus among urologists about whether to proceed with a radical prostatectomy if there is evidence of cancer spread to any of the lymph nodes. My point is simply that unless the lymph nodes are examined prior to removing the prostate gland the presence or absence of tumor in these lymph nodes cannot be known, and these lymph nodes are most readily examined when the retropubic surgical approach is used.

The recent popularization of laparascopic techniques in urology, however, has made it possible to remove the lymph nodes through four very small incisions in the abdomen (see Chapter 9); after obtaining frozen section reports on these nodes it is then feasible and reasonable to do the radical prostatectomy through the perineal approach.

The retropubic approach to the prostate for a radical prostatectomy is precisely the same as for the retropubic approach to BPH. A long up-and-down incision is made in the midline of the abdomen from the navel to the pubic bone. After the lymph nodes have been removed for study by the pathologist and a determination has been made to proceed with the removal of the prostate gland, the space underneath the pubic bone is cleaned and dissected and the removal of the entire prostate gland is generally begun at the end that is farthest from the bladder, next to the external urethral sphincter. The prostatic urethra is divided at this point; then it and the prostate gland through which it goes are pulled upwards toward the bladder while the dissection continues behind the prostate gland, separating it from the layer of tissue that is connected to the rectum on its other side. As the dissection continues between the prostate and the rectum, the seminal vesicles, which are behind the base of the bladder, come into view and will be removed along with the prostate gland. This dissection of the seminal vesicles from the back wall of the bladder is generally done after the bladder neck has been cut across. Once the seminal vesicles are free the entire prostate gland and the seminal vesicles are removed. The bladder neck is then stitched closed to a small enough diameter so that it is about the same size as the stump of the urethra from which the prostate was detached. The bladder neck is then pulled down into the pelvis and snugged up against the urethral stump and stitched to it. This stitching is done around a Foley catheter which has been inserted through the penis all the way into the bladder (Fig. 6–10).

The entire operation is a formidable one, generally taking between two and four hours. There is not infrequently a considerable loss of blood. Recovery from surgery is usually slower than from any of the forms of surgery that are done for BPH. The patient is generally in the hospital for about five days to a week and is then sent home with a catheter in place. The catheter is removed about three weeks postoperatively on a return visit.

The second, alternative surgical approach that is used for a radical prostatectomy is through the perineum, the area between the scrotum and the anus. This approach is called a radical perineal prostatectomy. Some surgeons who genuinely prefer the perineal route have come up with a method for removing and examining the pelvic lymph nodes. They explore and remove the retroperitoneal lymph nodes of the pelvis via the laparascopic approach; once the pathologist has come up with a frozen section report on those nodes, it is then feasible to carry out the second operation (the radical prostatectomy) via the perineal route. Using these two operations, the preferred surgical approach, for some urologists, via the

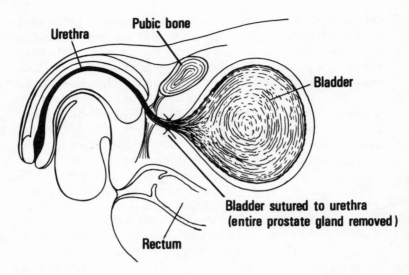

Figure 6–10 *Following a radical or total prostatectomy (removal of the prostate) by either the perineal or the retropublic approach, the bladder neck is sutured to the stump of the urethra. The entire prostate gland has been removed.*

perineum is combined with laparascopic removal of the lymph nodes to determine whether the urologist feels that the patient is potentially curable.

The reason that the perineal approach is favored by some urologists is because the postoperative course is much easier on a patient since an abdominal incision is considerably more uncomfortable that a perineal incision. Also, the exposure of the prostate gland and the actual surgical removal of the prostate are both somewhat easier with the perineal approach.

The surgical incision that is used for a radical perineal prostatectomy is usually in the shape of an inverted "U" going right over the anus, with the center of the U about three centimeters above the margin of the anus. In extending the incision deeply into the tissues of the perineum it is important to release the attachments of the rectum to the urethra so that the rectum will fall away towards the back of the patient while the urethra and ultimately the prostate gland are more anterior, thereby minimizing the chance of damaging the rectum. The prostate gland is freed from its surrounding structures by gentle dissection, and the urethra at the end of the prostate farthest from the bladder is isolated and divided. The bladder neck is freed from the prostate, and, once the prostate gland has been removed and the bladder neck has been closed sufficiently so that the size of its opening approximates the size of the urethral opening, the urethra and the bladder neck are stitched together. A catheter is left in place postoperatively for about two or three weeks.

Some Final Thoughts about Different Surgical Approaches

Should you be upset if your surgeon wants to do an open operation to relieve your BPH and you want him to do the operation transurethrally? I don't really think so, because the odds are very high that the urologist you have chosen is a thoroughly knowledgeable individual who knows as well as I do the pros and cons of the different surgical approaches. However, it is perfectly proper and reasonable for you to ask your urologist why he prefers the surgical approach that he has chosen. It is also proper to ask him as many other questions as you might have so that you will be completely satisfied with your urologic surgeon and with his planned operation. Assuming that you have confidence in your primary care physician who has referred you to this urologist, and assuming that your urologist is either board certified (by the American Board of Urology) or board eligible (he has taken the requisite training to be certified but has perhaps not been in practice quite long enough to be eligible to take the oral part of his certification examination), I think that you can feel comfortable with your urologist. However, you should always realize that there are many excellent urologists in this country, and if you are not happy, for whatever reason, with the individual to whom you have been referred then you should certainly feel free to ask your primary care physician to refer you to someone else. You should also never hesitate to ask your urologist if he or she is board certified or board eligible. Alternatively, you can look the urologist up in *Marquis' Directory of Medical Specialists* which is updated every other year.

Bilateral Orchiectomy (Removal of the Testes)

In the early 1940s it was conclusively demonstrated that the great majority (around 90 percent) of prostate cancers are dependent upon the male hormone (testosterone) for growth. This means that the growth and spread of prostate carcinoma (in 90 percent of patients) is enhanced by normal circulating blood levels of male hormone. More importantly, it means that the growth and spread of prostate carcinoma is markedly slowed by removal of the male hormone. It has long been known, because of this basic research on the influence of male hormones upon the spread of prostate cancer, that patients lived longer and with a better quality of life in the absence of any circulating testosterone. Although definitely not curative, the removal of the male hormone has been proven to significantly palliate patients with prostate cancer that has spread outside the confines of the prostate gland. The patients for whom removal of the male hormone might be considered beneficial are those patients in whom there is documented spread of cancer to the lymph nodes, to the bones, or elsewhere in the body.

Although there are several ways to reduce the circulating testosterone to near zero levels (see discussion in Chapter 5), removal of the testes (bilateral orchiectomy) has been considered for many years to be the most efficient way. Unfortunately, this operation is one that is understandably dreaded and feared by most men; for this reason it is often refused in favor of other procedures (hormonal therapy) which may not be as successful as bilateral orchiectomy in retarding the course of the cancer.

Many patients for whom bilateral orchiectomy is recommended are beyond the point of life where sexual intercourse is important. Regardless, what seems to be anathema to most men about bilateral orchiectomy is almost unrelated to intercourse itself and strikes at the very core of maleness: emasculation in an intellectual sense. Certainly this is the problem for most men who no longer are really interested in sexual intercourse. Bilateral orchiectomy, in and of itself, does not necessarily lead to impotence, and there are indeed men who continue to get erections after this operation. It does, however, lead to a loss of libido in most men. For those men who still want to pursue an active sex life there are several viable options (see Chapter 8).

The operation of bilateral orchiectomy is a very simple one that can be done under local or general anesthesia. A small incision, no more than one or two inches in length, is usually made in the middle portion of the lower part of the scrotum (between the two testes), and both testes can easily be removed through this one incision. Alternatively, some urologists like to make small incisions on each side of the scrotum through which the respective testes can be removed. The scrotum itself has relatively few pain fibers; so the postoperative course is marked by minimal discomfort, and the scrotal incision heals rapidly and well because of the normally excellent blood supply to the scrotum. Bilateral orchiectomy is such a relatively minor surgical procedure, in fact, that it can be done on an out-patient basis as well as the more traditional in-patient basis where a patient might stay in the hospital for a day or two following surgery.

Unfortunately, some urologists, accustomed to caring for patients with prostatic carcinoma, become quite callous to the mental trauma inflicted on a patient who is to be told that his testes need to be removed. Not infrequently, a more earthy form of language is used to tell the patient what needs to be done, and it is a rare man, indeed, who is not totally shattered by this news. Many urologists tend to be quite upset with patients who refuse the recommendation for this operation and opt instead for an alternative form of therapy. It has always been my policy to make a point of sitting down with my patient and trying to discuss this recommendation of bilateral orchiectomy in a very private setting and particularly in a very unhurried manner. I have found that most patients will ultimately go along with bilateral orchiectomy once they understand the shortcomings of alternative therapies and once they realize that their own self-image and self-worth are not totally contained in their testes. For those patients, however, who adamantly refuse orchiectomy, I will always seek an alternative means of treatment.

Radiation Therapy for Prostate Cancer

One of the time-honored, recognized, and widely-used forms for therapy of prostate cancer is radiation therapy. My own bias in favor of surgical treatment reflects, in part, the fact that I am a surgeon; but I would also like to think that it reflects my very genuine belief that the cure rate and long-term survival without any evidence of remaining cancer is significantly better with surgical treatment. Nevertheless, radiation therapy for prostate cancer is preferred and chosen by and for many patients; so a discussion of this treatment should be included.

There are two very different forms of radiation therapy currently being used in the United States. One form uses a lower voltage machine and is known as a cobalt unit. The other, higher voltage machine is know as a linear accelerator. This machine was developed in the 1940s, before the cobalt unit, but it was initially thought that its exceedingly high cost would relegate it to research and experimental use. The cobalt units therefore represented the initial type of equipment used in the modern era of radiation therapy in this country beginning in the mid-1950s. Technical advancements, however, made the linear accelerator a feasible method of delivering high-voltage radiation therapy to patients. Since about 1968 it has been the preferred method of delivering this form of therapy to cancer patients. The linear accelerator costs between one and one and a half million dollars per unit, and the cobalt unit costs about half that much. This cost differentiation represents the principal reason that cobalt units are still being used in some institutions around the country. The much higher voltage linear accelerators are able to deposit their radiation energy beneath the skin surface of the body so that skin damage, relatively common with cobalt units, is extremely uncommon with the linear accelerator. Moreover, the "scatter" or side effects from radiation to structures other than the target areas is also much less with the linear accelerators than with the cobalt units. Since the linear accelerator is the preferred type of equipment for the delivery of radiation therapy, further discussion will be limited to it.

Radiation therapy for patients with prostatic carcinoma, whether stage A, B, C, or D, is done daily (five times per week) for seven weeks. A total of 35 treatments are administered, with a total radiation dosage of between 6,500 and 7,000 rads (a rad is a unit of measurement of the amount of radiation received). For comparison purposes, the radiation therapy dosage for lung cancer is 5,000 to 6,000 rads; for colon cancer, it is 4,500 to 5,500 rads; and for cancer of the head and neck region it is 6,500 to 7,000 rads. Each of these 35 daily treatments takes about three minutes, and about half of the patients get short-term side effects (lasting for the duration of the treatment) of diarrhea usually requiring treatment with Lomotil. An occasional patient may have periodic flareups of diarrhea for years afterwards, but this is uncommon, and less than 1 percent of all patients will develop actual perforation of the large intestine or stricture of the large intestine. Other short-term side effects (during the duration of the therapy) may be loss of appetite, nausea, or, more commonly, the symptoms of cystitis which include frequency and urgency of the need to void. Additionally, about 50 percent of the patients having radiation therapy for prostate cancer become permanently impotent as a result of the therapy, although the mechanism for this impotency is not known. The long-term bladder effects of severe inflammation (cystitis) probably affect fewer than 10 percent of all patients. These will unquestionably be fewer in number when the radiation therapy is delivered by a therapist who is highly skilled in his craft, because there will then be less chance of structures other than the target structure (the prostate) being radiated.

The five-year survival statistics for radiation therapy run about 90 percent for stage A, to 80 percent for stage B, and 35 to 40 percent for stage C. These survival statistics are very similar to those found after radical surgery, but the principal difference, in my opinion, is that the survival after radical surgery is *without* any residual tumor whereas the survival after radiation therapy is very frequently *with* residual tumor. When the patients who have received radiation therapy are biopsied months and even several years after radiation therapy, over 50 percent of these patients show remaining cancer in the prostate gland. It is this finding that gives many urologists pause in recommending radiation therapy for those patients who would otherwise be suitable candidates for radical prostate surgery.

There is considerable controversy over the role of radiation therapy in stage D_1 prostate cancer patients. I feel, as do many, that once prostate cancer is in the lymph nodes, radiation therapy is not going to bring about a cure. There are some radiation therapists who disagree with this point of view and do indeed recommend that radiation therapy be done on both the lymph nodes and the prostate in those patients known to have stage D_1 cancer. The survival data for these stage D_1 patients, following radiation therapy, is poor and is not too different from that found with no treatment at all (other than bilateral orchiectomy).

In summary, radiation therapy unquestionably improves the survival of patients with prostate cancer from what it would be if those same patients had no treatment at all. In the best results reported, radiation therapy is comparable, in the short term (5 years) but not the long-term (10 and 15 years), to that offered by radical prostate surgery. But it must be remembered that this survival, following radiation therapy, is often *with* residual cancer remaining in the prostate gland. It must also be remembered that for those patients developing long-terms symptoms of urgency and frequency, these side effects can be disabling.

7

What You (the Patient) Can Anticipate at Each Step along the Way

If You Go to Your Doctor with Symptoms of Prostatic Inflammation or Infection

Probably the first, and perhaps the most important, thing that your doctor will do is to take a detailed medical history from you about your present symptoms, your past genitourinary tract symptoms or problems, and your health in general. All of this is very important in helping your doctor reach a correct diagnosis, and you should search your memory carefully and be honest about the answers you provide.

You will certainly be asked what specific problem or complaint brought you to the doctor. The answer to this is what physicians call the "chief complaint." Was it pain in the area between your scrotum and anus (the perineum)? Was it pain in your rectum? Was it pain or discomfort "deep inside" your penis? Have you had any sort of abnormal or unusual discharge from your penis? Have you had any burning or other discomfort during urination? Has your urine had a foul odor? Have you had fever accompanying your symptoms? Have you had pain anywhere else along with your symptoms? For how long have your present symptoms been bothering you? Have you ever before had any symptoms like the present ones? If so, how were you treated? Have you ever seen a urologist before for any of your present symptoms or similar ones? Have you ever had *any* other urologic complaints? Blood in your urine? Kidney stones? Any childhood history of urologic symptoms or disease?

Your physician will then ask you many questions pertaining to your sex life and your sexual history. This is extremely important so you should make every effort to be as honest and straightforward with your answers as possible. The reason your physician does this is because it is very common for men to come to a physician (particularly to a urologist) complaining of a genitourinary tract problem or symptom when the *real* reason the patient has come to the physician is because of a sexual problem. Most patients are reluctant to talk about their sexual problems, real or imagined. The astute physician realizes this and will ask questions during the course of the medical history to determine if indeed there is a sexual problem. You will be asked questions such as: Do you have any difficulty achieving erections? Are the erections sufficient for vaginal penetration? Are you able to keep your erections long enough to allow for vaginal penetration and orgasm? Is there anything at all about your sexual life that you would care to discuss?

Your physician will next ask you questions about your health in general, questions that are important for their own sake but could also impact on your specific urologic problem. Do you have diabetes or is there any family history of diabetes? Do you have high blood pressure, are you being treated for high blood pressure, or have you ever been treated for high blood pressure? Have you ever been told that you had tuberculosis or is there any history in your family of tuberculosis? Are you allergic to any medications? Are you allergic to anything of which you are aware? If so, what?

Your physician will next perform a physical examination, and the extent of the examination will depend in large measure on whether your physician is a primary care physician or a urologist. If the former, he will probably do a reasonably complete, albeit cursory, examination. If he is a urologist he will probably confine his examination to the genitourinary tract which is, after all, that part of the body related to the reason that you have come to see him. You will probably start the examination by lying down flat on your back on an examining table while your doctor quickly palpates your abdomen. This is simply to look for any lumps, bumps, or areas of pain or tenderness, or even an enlargement of your bladder which might suggest incomplete bladder emptying. He will next examine your genitals, usually while you are still lying on your back. This is important because it will enable your physician to determine the normalcy of your penis and testes. Remember that cancer of the testes is the most common form of solid cancer in males between the ages of 18 and 40, and it usually produces no symptoms at all. It is diagnosed only by a physical examination or by the patient doing a self-examination. Your physician will next ask you to stand up, at which time he will check you for a hernia in your groin area and for any abnormalities that might exist in your scrotum.

Now, considering the fact that you have come to the physician because of a set of symptoms which suggest that you either have inflammation or infection in your prostate gland or in your prostatic urethra (see Chapter 3), it is absolutely necessary that your physician determine with certainty if it is your prostate or your urethra that is the source of your difficulty. If it is your prostate, is it inflammation in that gland or is it infection? These questions are answered by a laboratory test of your urine. To do this your doctor will ask you to start to void into a sterile container that is marked #1. You will do this, putting perhaps an ounce or two of urine into the glass, and then, without stopping your urinary stream, you direct it out of glass #1 and briefly into the toilet before directing it into an empty sterile container marked #2. After voiding a couple of ounces of urine into this second glass, which will be the midstream urine, you will move glass #2 away from your urinary stream and void directly into the toilet, being certain to retain some urine in your bladder for what is to follow. Your physician will then do a digital rectal examination of your prostate and will "strip" or "massage" your prostate vigorously (see Chapter 2) so as to express secretions from the prostate gland into the prostatic urethra. During this time, you will grasp the end of your penis and keep it squeezed tightly shut so that none of the prostatic secretions escape during this prostatic massage. The prostatic stripping or massage is certainly not pleasant but neither is it painful and most patients feel that its worst aspect is the forceful feeling that some fluid (the prostatic fluid) is trying to come out of the urethra. In point of fact, there is often no fluid that comes out of the urethra at the conclusion of the prostatic massage; but if any does appear, it is collected for microscopic examination and culture. Most of the time the prostatic secretions have just pooled in the prostatic urethra, and to obtain them for examination you will be asked to void one more time into a glass marked #3. Into this container you will put an ounce or two of urine, which will then contain the secretions from the prostate gland. At this point you will simply finish emptying your bladder into the toilet.

It is the comparison between the number of bacteria in the three glasses of urine as well as the microscopic appearance of the prostatic secretions themselves (if any have been obtained) that will enable your doctor to tell you whether your symptoms are due to infection or inflammation in the prostate gland or infection in the urethra.

Once your doctor has determined whether your problem is in your urethra or your prostate he will be able to treat you. If the infection is in the prostatic portion of the urethra, where it will almost always be when there is a urethral infection (except for a gonorrheal infection), the drug of choice is tetracycline or one of its synthetic derivatives; therapy is usually continued for two or three weeks. If you have infection in your prostate gland (and this is very uncommon), the treatment will usually be with Bactrim or Septra (they are the same drug made by two different companies), geocillin, or one of the fluoroquinolones such as norfloxacin or ciprofloxacin, depending on the bacteria identified in the prostatic secretions. Treatment is usually necessary for at least a month and often for up to three months; but the treatment of chronic bacterial infection in the prostate is by no means always successful, and probably no more than one-half to two-thirds of patients with this problem actually achieve an eradication of the infection. The remaining patients may well have recurring infections over a period of many years. If you have a simple inflammation without any bacterial infection in your prostate your doctor may give you an antibiotic for one or two weeks, and you will be absolutely delighted when your physician additionally prescribes for you a program of frequent intercourse and / or masturbation. Inflammation of the prostate gland often results from inadequate, infrequent, and incomplete emptying of the prostate gland, and this is usually caused by a sudden diminution in the frequency of ejaculation. The treatment of this condition is therefore a singularly joyous one that most men appreciate greatly!

Some physicians tell patients who have infection or inflammation in the prostate that they should abstain from alcohol and any spicy or "hot" foods. The rationale for this is that these things, absorbed from the stomach into the bloodstream, may eventually reach the urine in concentrations high enough to cause a patient discomfort when the urine passes over the inflamed lining of the prostatic urethra. I do not agree at all with this thesis and I tell my patients that it is perfectly all right for them to eat or drink anything they want, and they will do no harm whatever to their prostate gland or prostatic urethra. However, I also tell my patients that if alcohol or any specific spicy or "hot" foods do cause them discomfort when they are urinating, then they might want to consider no longer using the things that cause the discomfort. It is up to the patient, however, to make this decision.

If You Go to Your Doctor with Symptoms of Benign Prostatic Hyperplasia (BPH)

You will probably go to see your doctor because you are getting up too many times at night to urinate, or you are urinating too frequently, or you feel you are not emptying your bladder, or you are wetting your pants after you think you have finished voiding. In any case, your doctor certainly will ask you many questions to confirm his very preliminary impression that you have BPH. The chances are that he would have this impression based only upon your presenting complaint and the fact that you are over 45 or 50 years of age. The older you are when you first see your physician with these complaints, the more likely he will be to think that your diagnosis is BPH.

Nevertheless, your physician will undoubtedly ask you many questions, all of which are designed to confirm his initial impression that BPH is your problem. How many times do you get up at night? Do you have trouble starting your urinary stream? Does your urinary stream ever stop completely before you finish voiding and then start up again some seconds later? Do you feel as if you empty your bladder when you void? Is your urinary stream noticeably weaker than it was five years ago? Have you ever had any pain or discomfort or burning while urinating? When you get the urge to urinate do you have to do it right away or can you wait until a convenient time presents itself? Have you ever lost any urine involuntarily? Have you ever seen any blood in your urine? All of these questions will help your doctor to diagnose BPH since all these symptoms are associated with this condition.

There are, however, other conditions which will enter your physician's mind when he listens to your litany of symptoms. Some of the conditions which must be differentiated from BPH are scarring in your urethra, an abnormal contraction of your bladder neck, and nerve damage to your bladder so that it does not function normally. The urethral scarring is usually due to an old gonorrhea infection or some sort of injury that has been done to the urethra in the past that led to the scar. A careful history can usually determine whether or not urethral scarring is a viable alternative diagnosis based on the duration of the symptoms. If you have not had any symptoms of voiding difficulty until the relatively recent past and nothing has transpired that could have led to a urethral scar, then that possible diagnosis is obviously not a tenable one. Similarly, a bladder neck contraction, unless it has followed a previous operation on the prostate, would have been present since a very early age and the history of voiding difficulty would go back for many years. Finally, nerve damage to the bladder is not very common, although it certainly is a distinct possibility if you have diabetes or have had any sort of spinal cord injury or major surgery in the area of your pelvis. A neurogenic bladder is the term used when there is nerve damage to the bladder. It simply means a bladder that has abnormal innervation or abnormal musculature. This abnormality can lead to symptoms that are readily confused with those of BPH; but neurogenic bladders are not very common as compared with BPH, and so the initial diagnosis for a patient with the symptoms noted above must be BPH.

The physical examination starts with the abdomen, and a particular emphasis is placed on looking for an enlarged or distended bladder since this finding would go along with BPH. The digital rectal examination helps to estimate the size of the prostate gland, and therefore of the BPH enlargement. It also is done to be sure that there are no hard or firm areas on the prostate that might be suggestive of malignancy. What your doctor is *not* able to do on a digital rectal examination of the prostate is to state unequivocally that you do or do not have BPH that is responsible for your symptoms. This is because a normal-sized prostate can still result in profound obstruction to the flow of urine. The obstruction would be due to an enlarged middle lobe of the prostate, which cannot be palpated on digital rectal examination, but which is the most common cause of the symptoms of BPH. Also, even if the prostate gland were noticeably enlarged this would only be suggestive, and not confirmatory, of lateral-lobe enlargement that is encroaching upon the prostatic urethra and hindering the flow of urine (see Chapter 4 for a detailed discussion of BPH).

Another extremely important reason for doing the digital rectal examination is to perform a test that will tell your physician whether you may have a neurogenic bladder (a bladder with less than normal innervation). Your physician will briskly squeeze the head of your penis while his finger is in your rectum, and a normal and positive reflex will result in a contraction of your anal sphincter on his finger. The absence of this anal sphincter contraction does not necessarily signify that a neurogenic bladder is present but it certainly will lead your physician to consider that possibility since it is a condition that must be differentiated from BPH.

A urine analysis is usually done at this point, primarily to look for white blood cells (pus cells) which might possibly indicate the presence of infection in the urine. If white cells are present the urine should be cultured, and if there is any suggestion of past or present history of urinary tract infection the urine should probably be cultured.

Blood is obtained from a vein in your arm for creatinine and blood urea nitrogen levels (see Chapter 2), in order to evaluate your kidney function. A blood prostate specific antigen level is done as well, and if it is elevated it *may* indicate the presence of prostate cancer. The presence of prostate cancer would in many cases have been suggested by the digital rectal examination; but in 25 percent or more of patients having prostate cancer the rectal examination will suggest an entirely benign gland even though there is cancer inside it (see Chapter 5, stage A) that may or may not have already spread beyond the confines of the prostate.

You will recall from Chapter 4 that there are two broad sets of indications, subjective and objective, for prostate surgery to relieve BPH. First, surgery may be indicated when a patient's symptoms of bladder outlet obstruction are bothersome enough that he would like relief from them. Second, surgery is probably necessary when there is definite objective evidence of an inability to empty the bladder, back pressure on the kidneys, or deteriorating kidney function. To evaluate the second broad category of indications for surgery, your doctor will perform several studies, including an evaluation of your kidneys to see if there is a significant back pressure upon them due to incomplete bladder emptying. This determination is usually done with an x-ray study that is called an excretory urogram (see Chapter 2). If you tell your doctor that you have moderate symptoms of difficulty voiding but you are concerned about whether or not you need prostate surgery, the doctor will realize that your symptoms alone do not warrant surgery but that it is important to be certain that you are not slowly damaging your kidneys because of back pressure on them from an incompletely emptied bladder. An excretory urogram will show if there is any such back pressure and it will also show how well you empty your bladder. The same information can be learned from an ultrasound study of the kidneys combined with a kidney and bladder scan (see Chapter 2). These alternative studies are preferable if there is any question of an allergic type of reaction to an injected contrast medium that may have been used in the past.

Based upon the history you have given to your physician, the physical examination, and the excretory urogram (or alternative tests) that has been done, your doctor now feels that it is quite likely that you do indeed have obstruction to your flow of urine from an enlargement of your prostate gland. At this point, your physician may want to do one or both of two additional studies; whether these are done will often depend on how certain your doctor is of the diagnosis of BPH. If, for example, you are a patient who has been followed for a long time while your symptoms of bladder outlet obstruction have gradually worsened, your doctor very likely may not feel the need to do any other studies before suggesting that you have prostate surgery. On the other hand, if you are a new patient who is being seen for the first time, your doctor may feel that other studies such as a voiding flow rate or a cystoscopic exam, or both, should be done. The voiding flow rate is really a very simple test which measures the number of milliliters per second that you are able to void into a container when you are voiding at your peak or maximum flow rate. Although there are sophisticated machines that are used to measure this, it is often done quite adequately by having you start to void into a toilet and then, when you feel that your urine is flowing at its peak or maximum (without straining), directing the flow into a measured container while your doctor or a technician starts a stopwatch. When you feel your urinary flow begin to slow and taper off you direct your stream back into the toilet and the stopwatch is stopped. The number of milliliters of urine per second that you produced when your flow was at its maximum is your peak urinary flow rate. If this is under 10 ml / second you probably need surgical relief of your prostatic obstruction. If it is over 20 ml / second you probably do not need any surgery. If it is somewhere in between, the decision of whether to operate on your prostate gland will be based on your physician's overall impression of your problem and an analysis of all of the objective data that have been compiled. In borderline cases, I generally prefer to defer surgery.

The cystoscopic examination is the *sine qua non* for many urologists in making the diagnosis of BPH because it permits an actual look at the existing obstruction to the flow of urine. The cystoscopic exam also permits the simultaneous and very accurate measurement of residual urine. It is my practice to always have a patient void immediately prior to cystoscopy; when the cystoscope is introduced into the bladder any urine that is inside comes out through the cystoscope where it can be collected and measured. Residual urine (the amount of urine left in the bladder following voiding) should ideally be 0 ml; the more residual urine there is in a patient with BPH the greater the need for surgical treatment. I generally do not get too excited about residual urine until it is 100 ml or so. Increasing amounts beyond that, and particularly far beyond that, pretty well mandate prostate surgery.

The cystoscopic examination itself is done with an instrument about as big around as a ballpoint pen with a light and a lens on one end and a viewing lens on the other end (see Fig. 2–10). After the urethra is well anesthetized using an anesthetic jelly squirted into it, the instrument is introduced into the urethral opening at the end of the penis and very slowly and gently advanced up through the penile urethra, the prostatic urethra, and finally into the bladder. When it is in the prostatic urethra, and the light and lens are about at the level of the external urethral sphincter, the physician can accurately estimate the amount of obstructing prostatic tissue and the degree to which the BPH is actually obstructing the flow of urine. However, it must be emphasized that the only thing the urologist is really able to see is the extent of *anatomic* obstruction. The cystoscopic exam is unable to reveal very much about the *functional* obstruction. In other words, the urethra that appears to be quite severely obstructed by BPH tissue may in fact offer minimal resistance to the flow of urine and such patients may have little or no need for surgery. On the other hand, what appears to be a relatively modest degree of obstruction can severely impede the flow of urine in some patients. The cystoscopic exam is often not carried out in the office in those patients for whom the physician feels that surgery is definitely indicated because the cystoscopic exam, although very important, should not alone be the determining factor in whether surgery is done. I personally limit my office cystoscopic exam to those patients for whom I feel that surgery is probably *not* indicated, but for whom I want to get a "base line" idea of the degree of prostatic obstruction in order to give the patient a rough idea about if or when prostatic surgery might be needed in the future. For that group of patients for whom surgery *is* recommended, I generally carry out the cystoscopic exam on the operating table, under a spinal or general anesthestic, immediately before proceeding with the operation itself. The purpose of the cystoscopy at this time is twofold: to evaluate the interior of the bladder to make sure that there are no unexpected diseases in the bladder requiring treatment, and to get as good an idea as possible about the size of the obstructing prostatic tissue which is estimated with the cystoscope in the bladder and an examining finger in the rectum. In this fashion I am able to estimate the amount of BPH tissue that is between the cystoscope and the rectal finger.

The cystoscopic exam, when it is done as an office procedure, could not be called pleasant or totally without discomfort; but it certainly is not a painful exam as long as local anesthestic is used and the urologist is gentle and skilled.

For a cystoscopic exam in the doctor's office, you will be placed on an examining table with your legs spread wide apart and supports placed behind your knees to hold them in an elevated position. This is known as the lithotomy position and is very similar to the position in which a woman is placed when she is about to give birth. Your genitals will be washed with soap and water and perhaps with a disinfectant or antiseptic solution. A local anesthestic, usually in jelly form, will then be squirted into your urethra, and it ideally is supposed to go all the way down the urethra and into the bladder. The local anesthetic that I use is a jelly that comes out of a tube that looks very much like a toothpaste tube, and the little nozzle on the end of the tube is inserted into the opening at the end of the penis. The tube itself is then briskly squeezed, forcing the jelly down into the urethra. To some patients, this is the most unpleasant part of the entire procedure. After allowing three to five minutes for the anesthetic to work, the cystoscope is inserted into the urethra and very gently advanced into the bladder. When the instrument is in place you should not feel any pain but you will be aware of the sensation that something is inside you. Your urologist will probably take between two and five minutes for the entire procedure, and will use two different lenses to examine you. One of these is a right-angle lens that enables the urologist to examine the interior of the bladder. The other lens is known as a foroblique lens, a "straight-ahead" lens that enables the urologist to examine the prostatic urethra. I have not found it necessary to use any injectable tranquilizers or pain killers to facilitate cystoscopy, although some urologists do use these. My concern is simply that when such medications are used it is generally not safe for the patient to drive his car for several hours.

When all of the above studies, or as many of them as the urologist deems are indicated, have been finished and the evidence points to the need for prostate surgery, the question invariably comes up: "How soon?" There is usually a good bit of leeway here and you should frankly discuss your desires and feelings with your physician. If the indications for surgery consist only of the symptoms that you have when you void, I feel that you as the patient should make the decision as to when you want the surgery. It is my practice never to push or urge a patient to have surgery sooner than he desires it as long as the indications for surgery are limited to the patient's own voiding problems.

On the other hand, there are certain objective findings that I feel remove the timing of surgery from the wishes of the patient because in such cases the indications for surgery really have nothing to do with a patient's symptoms. These objective findings are those which, if not reversed, can well lead to kidney damage, recurring infection, an acute inability to void, or even uremic poisoning. Once a patient has a residual urine that is over 100 cc, or possibly even 150 cc, surgery should be seriously considered. The need for it becomes more pressing as the amount of residual urine increases, because of the risk of back pressure on the kidneys from increasing amounts of residual urine. Once a patient has had one episode of bladder infection I feel that it is inevitable that other infections will follow unless the residual urine that predisposes the patient to bladder infections is eliminated. Once the excretory urogram shows obstruction to the drainage of one or both kidneys, surgical relief is indicated because, if left untreated, irreversible renal damage and / or renal failure may occur. Therefore, if you have any of these objective findings including recurrent infection, high residual urine, x-ray evidence of back pressure on your kidneys, or an elevated serum creatinine (which indicates kidney damage), the timing of surgery is no longer elective but should be carried out as soon as possible. Certainly, surgery in any case is not an emergency as it is with acute appendicitis, but a general rule of thumb is that when there are objective indications for prostate surgery it should be done at the very earliest time that is possible for both the patient and his physician.

Once a decision has been made to proceed with prostate surgery for the relief of BPH you will often feel a sense of relief because you have made the decision to go ahead and you know that your bothersome symptoms of prostate disease will soon be a thing of the past. The results of surgery for prostatic obstruction are really quite excellent and the vast majority of patients find it not at all unpleasant and almost "a breeze."

After you have been admitted to the hospital you will have a general physical examination to assess your overall condition. This is usually done by your family physician or internist, but it may also be done by a resident physician or your own urologist. You will probably also have a chest x-ray and an electrocardiogram as well as basic laboratory blood work and urine tests prior to surgery. An anesthesiologist will probably visit you the night before surgery to discuss your choice of anesthesia, and you should share with the anesthesiologist your preferences and any fears or concerns you may have. In this cost-conscious era, many patients having a TURP are admitted to the hospital on the morning of surgery and see the anesthesiologist on that morning. The general physical exam and laboratory studies are done prior to hospitalization. Most urologists prefer a spinal anesthetic to one that puts the patient to sleep, and the reasons for this are twofold. First, the muscles of the lower abdomen and the pelvic floor are usually more relaxed with a spinal anesthetic; second, there are none of the lung complications with a spinal anesthetic that sometimes are present after a general or inhalational anesthetic. Some patients develop a collapse of small segments of the lung; other patients may develop a pneumonia in some portions of the lung. Although these are invariably treated successfully, the fact remains that with spinal anesthesia these findings virtually never occur. There are certain reasons the anesthesiologist may have for *not* wanting to perform spinal anesthesia. Two of these are previous spinal surgery or spinal injury and certain types of cardiovascular disease that do not tolerate drops in blood pressure which frequently accompany spinal anesthesia.

During the surgery itself you will not be at all uncomfortable regardless of the surgical approach that is taken. You will feel absolutely nothing if you have had a spinal anesthetic and you will of course be asleep and therefore feel absolutely nothing if you are given a general or inhalational anesthetic. The operation itself will take anywhere from one to two hours, regardless of the surgical approach. When it is finished you will be in the recovery room, a special area where patients can be watched extraordinarily closely by highly trained nursing personnel as well as anesthesiologists, while they recover from the effects of the anesthesia and while they are in the immediate postoperative period.

If your prostate surgery has been done via the transurethral route you will have one tube (catheter) in your bladder following surgery. This will be a catheter that will be placed through the penis and into the bladder. The catheter stays in place because of an inflatable bag that is larger than the size of the bladder neck (see Fig. 2–9) thereby preventing it from slipping out of the bladder. For the first day or two following surgery you may have a continuous flow of an irrigating solution running into your bladder through a side channel in the catheter and then returning, mixed with the urine and blood that is normally in the bladder following surgery, through the regular catheter channel that is used to drain the bladder. The purpose of this irrigation is to prevent clot formation and plugging up of the catheter. There is usually a certain amount of bleeding from the area of the prostatic urethra where the surgery is done; it is this bleeding which at times can cause the catheter to obstruct because of clots. Usually, by the day after surgery, or sometimes the following day, it is possible to discontinue the continuous bladder irrigation; by the second or third day following surgery, the regular urine drainage from the bladder will generally be clear of visible blood. When it is clear, your physician may remove the catheter. I generally do this on the second or third day following surgery, with my patient leaving the hospital later that same day or on the next day.

During these few days in the hospital, you will have almost no discomfort and certainly no pain. Some patients do occasionally suffer from bladder spasms, which are usually due to the pressure of the inflatable catheter bag touching the very sensitive bladder trigone. These spasms can almost always be relieved or prevented by rectal suppositories of belladonna and opium which act directly on the bladder to relax it. It is uncommon for a patient to require an injectable narcotic for postoperative pain, and by the evening of the surgery or the next morning you will most likely be eating and drinking food and fluids as desired and walking around your room or in the corridors of the hospital carrying the drainage bag into which your catheter drains. The intravenous tubing to which you will be attached during surgery and immediately afterwards is usually disconnected and removed by the night of surgery or the next morning, once you have begun to drink fluids and to eat.

If you have had your prostate surgery done by one of the open approaches (the suprapubic or retropubic approach, see

Chapter 6), you will undoubtedly have considerable pain and discomfort when your anesthesia (either spinal or general) wears off because the incision in your abdomen will be painful. The pain will be helped greatly by injections of whichever narcotic your doctor has prescribed; but you must remember that most nurses will not give you any narcotic for pain unless you specifically request it. In many hospitals a new method of delivering narcotic relief for pain to postoperative patients is now in place. This is referred to as Patient Controlled Analgesia. It consists of a machine that automatically monitors whatever narcotic is placed into it (usually morphine); so whenever you push a button that is at your bedside, a small dose of the narcotic leaves the machine and goes into the tubing that is providing you with your intravenous fluids. A lockout mechanism prevents you from overdosing yourself with the narcotic, and the amount that you receive with each push of the button combined with the fact that you are able to receive the narcotic virtually whenever you want it lead to a smooth and relatively pain-free postoperative period. With the older, but still very much in use, method of the patient having to ring for the nurse in order to get a narcotic shot it is rather more the rule than the exception that the bell will not be answered promptly and, even if it is, the narcotic will not be delivered promptly. Consequently the patient's pain gets to a nearly intolerable point by the time the injection is given. It is very interesting to note that in hospitals that have switched to the Patient Controlled Analgesia machines the total dose of narcotic received by each patient is actually less than the total narcotic dose received when it is being given in isolated injections by the floor nurses.

If you have a suprapubic approach to your prostate you will have a tube coming out of your lower abdomen that goes straight into your bladder. This is in addition to the bladder catheter that is in your penis. If you have had a retropubic approach you will only have one bladder catheter and that will be the one in your penis. The abdominal incisions and the pain from them are the same with either the suprapubic or the retropubic routes. When open surgery has been done the catheters (either one or both) are allowed to drain freely by gravity drainage rather than with continuous irrigation. This is because during an open operation either the bladder or the true prostate capsule has been opened; and if continuous irrigation were used and the outflow catheter should accidentally become plugged with a clot, the bladder or the true capsule of the prostate might be forceably reopened by the resulting large collection of fluid in the bladder. With either of the open operations you will probably require narcotics for several days postoperatively and will be in the hospital for about seven to ten days after surgery. Some patients begin to drink fluids and to eat a soft diet the day after surgery, but most patients who have an open type of prostatectomy are really not eating very much until the third or fourth day following surgery.

Many men are seriously concerned about the consequences, emotional or physical, of not moving their bowels on a daily basis. Following prostate surgery your doctor actually will not want you to move your bowels for three or four days, at least, and this is particularly true if your stools have a tendency to be particularly firm. This is because there is only a thin bit of connecting tissue between the rectum and the true capsule and true prostate tissue that normally remains behind after an operation for BPH. The pressure of a very hard stool pressing against the true prostate gland so near the area from which the BPH was removed could stir up a considerable amount of bleeding from the site of the surgery. For the same reason it is extremely important that patients, during their hospital convalescence and for at least three weeks afterwards, absolutely not strain at stool; this is best accomplished if a stool softener such as Metamucil is used.

The great majority of patients who have prostate surgery have uninfected urine prior to surgery. Nevertheless there are many physicians who feel more comfortable putting their patients on prophylactic antibiotics a day or two before surgery, and continuing this through the hospitalization and for anywhere from two to six weeks postoperatively. It is my practice, however, not to use antibiotics unless there is a preoperative infection or unless the patient is in a high risk group for infections, such as a diabetic patient or one who is on steroids. Should an infection occur during the convalescence then antibiotics are of course used. But recall from an earlier chapter that the many white blood cells present in the urine during the first two or three months following surgery are *not* necessarily an indication of infection, but only of the normal healing process that follows prostate surgery.

Any major surgical procedure, including prostate surgery, takes a lot more out of a patient than he may realize. You will find that it takes about three months following surgery before you will begin to feel like your old self again in terms of vigor, vitality, and a get-up-and-go feeling. During this convalescence you should realize that the prostatic urethra, where the surgery was done, will not be totally healed with a new lining for about three months following surgery; and if you have an open operation the muscles of your abdominal wall are not healed firmly for about six weeks postoperatively. Therefore, for at least six weeks after any kind of open prostate surgery, you should avoid intense physical exercise that could cause a disruption of the abdominal wound before all of the layers are firmly healed. For a similar length of time you would be well advised to avoid any vigorous exercise and particularly any straining, lifting, or heavy work that could possibly result in bleeding from the actual site of the prostatic surgery. After about six weeks, even though the area of the surgical procedure has not yet healed completely, the risk of bleeding or any other complication is very minimal and patients are generally free to do whatever they choose, including a resumption of any sexual activities. I do, however, strongly advise my patients against doing any sort of housework for a minimum of five years!

Up until the time that the inside of the prostate gland is completely healed with its new lining, it is certainly possible that you may have some voiding discomfort and perhaps some frequency or urgency; you will probably have some nocturia as well. However, you will undoubtedly notice that your urinary stream is a strong one and it should be just about as large in caliber as your stream used to be when you were 20 years old! If you have a lot of frequency, though, you will be voiding often and in relatively small amounts, and so you may not always notice the good caliber and strength of your stream. When your bladder is full (at least 200 ml), you will indeed realize the formidable size and force of your urinary stream. As the area inside your prostate gland heals, any frequency, urgency, or burning on urination will gradually subside, although the nocturia may persist indefinitely. Getting up once or twice each night may well be nothing more than a residual habit from the years that you did this prior to your surgery, and this habit may remain forever. It does *not* mean that your surgery was unsuccessful.

I usually have my postoperative patients return to the office for followup care about two weeks after leaving the hospital, four to six weeks after that, and then again about six months postoperatively. These visits are made so that the patient's progress in a normal and satisfactory manner can be verified and also to check the patient's urine to make sure that there is no infection in it. I further recommend to my patients that they return annually thereafter. This is primarily so that I can do a digital rectal examination of the prostate, as well as a blood prostate specific antigen (PSA) test, to try to detect any possible early findings suggestive of prostate cancer, because, as will be remembered, the operation for BPH leaves behind the true prostate tissue which is the tissue in which prostate cancer originates.

A return to normal sexual activity is usually a relatively high priority for most patients; this should probably be deferred until the operative site is entirely healed, although it is not necessary to wait until the prostatic urethra has an entirely new lining. Within four to six weeks after surgery it is safe to resume full and normal sexual activity. Probably the only reason for not doing this any earlier is that the spasmodic contractions that occur in the prostatic urethra at the time of ejaculation could trigger delayed bleeding. Once six weeks or so have passed following surgery, the risk of a delayed bleed is very slight. From this time until the prostatic urethra is completely relined with normal mucosa the only "risk" of intercourse is that there may be some discomfort at the time of ejaculation because the area going into spasm has not as yet healed completely. As a general rule, those patients who

achieved full and normal erections preoperatively can anticipate the return of these erections postoperatively any time
after the catheter has been removed or within the first two to
three weeks following surgery.

If Your Doctor Finds That
You Have Prostatic Cancer

There can't be many words in the human language that
are as fearsome as cancer. If your doctor should find it necessary to tell you that you have cancer in your prostate gland
it is particularly fearsome because you are absolutely certain
that you will be impotent before long, and you will never again
enjoy sexual intercourse. When you first go to your physician
the chances are good that you will not have any urinary tract
complaints at all but will really be going for a routine physical
examination. Alternatively, you may go to your physician for
some totally unrelated problem such as a pain in your elbow
or your shoulder, and when your physician takes the opportunity to do a thorough physical exam he finds to his surprise
and to your horror that there is a suspicious, firm area that
he has palpated on your prostate while doing a digital rectal
examination. You will undoubtedly be referred to a urologist
who will surely repeat the digital rectal examination to form
an independent opinion about the suspicious area on your
prostate. Blood tests consisting of a prostate specific antigen
and possibly an acid phosphatase level as well will probably be
ordered (see Chapter 2). If the urologist also feels that the
lesion is suspicious it will be biopsied, probably in the office
but possibly in the hospital. This is not at all painful since the
action of the biopsy "gun" is so rapid that the biopsy itself is
virtually painless. Your urologist will quite likely use an ultrasound probe to examine your prostate and he will very likely
do the biopsy of your prostate using ultrasound to guide the
biopsy needle into the suspicious part of your prostate. The
ultrasound probe used for prostate examinations is about twice
the size of an ordinary lead pencil and it is usually done when
you are in a lying down position. It is not painful.

If the biopsy suggests that you do indeed have prostatic cancer the first thing your physician will probably want to do is obtain certain tests, on an outpatient basis, that will determine the likelihood that the cancer is still confined within your prostate gland and therefore probably curable.

Your doctor may next want to obtain bone x-rays, abdominal CT scans, and bone scans to confirm that there is no suggestion of cancer spread to any bones or lymph nodes. All of the foregoing tests are referred to as staging the cancer to determine the stage of the cancer at the time that it is discovered and treatment is contemplated (see Chapter 5). Staging determines if the cancer is still confined within your prostate gland or if it has spread outside of the prostate. Your urologist will probably then discuss with you the various treatment options. His recommendations will undoubtedly be dependent upon whether your cancer is still confined within the prostate gland (although this cannot be determined with absolute certainty until the lymph nodes of the pelvis are removed surgically and examined microscopically) as well as his own philosophy about the role of radiation therapy in treating cancer of the prostate and about whether he feels that aggressive therapy is still justified in the presence of demonstrated cancer in the lymph nodes (see Chapters 5 and 6).

If the option of radiation therapy is to be recommended, a patient is usually referred to a radiation therapist who is a specialist in this branch of medicine. Although radiation therapy is a thoroughly accepted and acceptable alternative to the surgical treatment of prostate cancer, I do not believe it to be as good, and I only recommend it for those patients whose general medical health will not allow a major surgical procedure or who, for other reasons, choose not to undergo any surgical procedure (see Chapters 5 and 6 for a more detailed discussion of radiation therapy). Still another treatment option is the placing of radioactive "seeds" directly into the prostate gland at the time of surgery after the lymph nodes have been examined and found to be negative. This form of treatment has achieved considerable popularity in the past, but even its strongest adherents are no longer recommending it because the results are no better than they are with external, standard radiation therapy and because its complications have been considerable (primarily consisting of unpleasant radiation effects on the rectum and bladder). A newer form of "seed" implantation has considerable promise but the long-term results remain to be proven. This method—brachytherapy—places many seeds into the prostate under ultrasound guidance for greater accuracy, and these seeds are removed after three days. This is combined with conventional external beam radiation therapy.

Assuming you choose to "go for the cure" with a radical prostatectomy, you will be hospitalized and given cleansing enemas as well as a bowel prep. This is a regime of oral solutions intended to sterilize the intestinal contents as much as possible, because sometimes the rectum is inadvertently opened during the course of a radical prostatectomy. This is not generally of any serious consequence and it can easily be repaired, but it can be a problem if the bowel has not been properly cleansed and sterilized prior to the intestinal injury.

The radical prostatectomy itself is a formidable operation (see Chapter 6) that will probably take between two and four hours, including the removal and examination of the lymph nodes of the pelvis and the radical or total prostatectomy. Following surgery there is generally only one bladder catheter and it goes through the penis. There are generally some drains left in the lower part of the abdomen that come out to the skin so that any amount of delayed bleeding and urine leakage can also come out and not collect down in the pelvis. These drains remain inside you for several days or until there is no more drainage. Removal of the drains is not painful. You will be in pain postoperatively but the pain will be no worse than if you had one of the open types of prostate surgery for the removal of BPH. However, because of the length of the operation and because the intestines are often handled during the surgery, there is often a marked slowing down of the normal intestinal contractions for a short period of time. A tube is therefore sometimes placed through your nose and into your stomach and connected to a gentle suction machine, so that the fluids that would accumulate because of the lack of normal stomach and intestinal contractions can be sucked out through the tube rather than left to accumulate where they might cause a big swelling of the abdomen. This tube, if used, is usually left in place after a radical prostatectomy for three or four days or until your own intestinal contractions begin to work normally and you are able to pass flatus (gas), a sure sign that intestinal activity has returned to normal. Once the tube is removed, you will be able to eat normally. By the day after surgery you will probably be able to sit up in a chair and will, hopefully, be able to take a brief walk, the duration of which will increase each day. Without any doubt, you will have a certain amount of pain and discomfort from this surgery that will require narcotics for its relief. If your hospital is able to give you one of the Patient Controlled Analgesia machines (see above), any postoperative pain and discomfort you might have will be enormously minimized.

The Foley catheter that was placed into your bladder at the time of surgery serves both to drain the bladder during the period of healing and as a splint around which the area where the bladder neck was stitched to the stump of the ure-thra can heal. I generally like to leave this catheter in place for about three weeks after surgery. The presence of the catheter serves to minimize any urine leakage from the area of the repair which might occur since it is extremely difficult to actually do a watertight repair. It is my practice to send patients home from the hospital, following radical prostatec-tomy, after five days to one week, and to see the patient as an outpatient in order to remove the catheter about three weeks from the time of hospital discharge.

When the catheter is removed, most patients will not have total control of urinary continence, and at first will leak urine to a greater or lesser degree for at least a few days. For this reason a patient is usually given a number of pads that can go inside his shorts to protect his clothing. Within a short period of time, the vast majority of patients recover their continence to the degree that there is not a constant leak while walking around. However, a certain degree of incontinence may remain for several weeks or even months while the entire continence mechanism improves gradually. So the vast majority of patients have little trouble with urinary leakage within the time frame of three weeks to three months after surgery. The degree of continence will continue to improve for up to six months or a year after surgery; but if leakage of urine still persists beyond a year it will probably require definitive therapy (see Chapter 8).

The period of convalescence following radical prostate surgery may take longer than the period following surgery for BPH. This is simply because the surgical procedure itself takes much longer and is much more traumatizing to the patient. Within three or four months you should be feeling as well as you were prior to surgery and able to do all the things that you could do prior to surgery. Obviously, with some individuals the time for a full recuperation can be even longer but this is determined more by the individual than by any variations in the operative procedure.

Many patients want to know about the resumption of sexual activities following radical prostatectomy and particularly if they are going to be able to achieve erections. As a general rule, it is probably fair and safe to say that if erections are going to return following radical prostate surgery, they may take up to six months or even a year to do so. Prior to this time one just cannot say whether or not potency will be present. In any case, the operative site is well healed within six weeks following surgery; so sexual activity could safely be resumed at any time after that point if erections are present. When radical prostatectomy is carried out, it is sometimes possible to avoid damaging the nerves on both sides of the prostate gland that control erection. Depending on the location of the prostate cancer and its size, it may well be possible to spare one or both of these nerves that control erection. If they are both spared, a patient will maintain at least partial potency following a radical prostatectomy. If one of them is spared, a patient may still maintain some potency. If neither nerve is spared, a patient will probably not maintain potency. In any case, even if potency is preserved, there will not be any ejaculate at the time of orgasm because the prostate and seminal vesicles have been removed, and the vasa have been tied off because there is no place for any sperm to go once the prostate and seminal vesicles have been removed. For those patients who are not able to achieve erections within six months to a year following surgery the option of treatment with one of the newer forms of penile prostheses or with penile injections is a very viable one and one which is chosen by many patients (see Chapter 8).

Although not generally of any concern to a man having a radical prostectomy for cancer of the prostate, I should probably note that these patients are permanently infertile following this operation. This is because removal of the entire prostate gland, including the prostatic urethra, precludes having any place for the spermatozoa to be deposited. Recall that the spermatozoa usually enter the prostatic urethra through the ejaculatory ducts (see Fig. 1–3). As part of the surgical procedure, therefore, the vas deferens are simply tied off.

8

Complications
of Prostate Surgery

Surgery for Benign Disease (BPH)

Since the vast majority of operations on the prostate for the
relief of benign prostatic hyperplasia are done via the transurethral route, complications of surgery for BPH will be discussed primarily as they relate to the transurethral approach.
However, the same complications can occur when one of the
open forms of surgical approach is used.

Postoperative Bleeding. As a general rule the sometimes
extensive bleeding that can occur during the course of prostatic surgery is completely controlled by the end of the operation, and the bleeding that occurs during the first two or
three days after surgery is minimal. The urine is usually clear
of all visible bleeding by the third or fourth postoperative day,
although microscopic blood will normally persist in the urine
for two to three months.

There is, however, really no way to clamp and tie blood
vessels within the prostatic urethra during the operation
because of the limited access to the area. Therefore when the

transurethral approach to surgery is used, bleeding vessels are cauterized or fulgurated with the same surgical instrument that is used to trim away the prostate gland. This leads to a scab forming as a seal over the blood vessel in much the same fashion that a scab will form on a knee that has been cut. Normally, the scab will fall off two or three weeks following surgery, and by that time the blood vessel is healed. However, about 1 percent of the patients who have prostate surgery may have a premature falling off of one or more of the scabs that cover a blood vessel. This may lead to bleeding which can at times be quite brisk. In my experience the principal cause for this sort of delayed bleeding is a patient straining at stool, and I find that it is worth taking the time to explain this to a patient convalescing from surgery. Patient cooperation and the use of a stool softener for two or three weeks postoperatively will usually prevent this complication. In any case, if delayed bleeding does occur a patient can help himself by drinking plenty of fluids so as to make a lot of urine and "wash out" the blood, although at times the bleeding is severe enough to require re-admission to the hospital. If this happens the bleeding can usually be controlled simply by inserting a Foley catheter into the bladder for a day or two. The pressure of the catheter on the bleeding blood vessel within the urethra usually serves to stop the bleeding. On infrequent occasions, it is necessary to cystoscope the patient under anesthesia in order to cauterize or fulgurate the bleeding vessel.

Incontinence. Incontinence is probably the most feared and the most distressing complication of prostate surgery for both the patient and the physician. The patient is extremely unhappy for the obvious reason that he cannot control his urine, and the physician is equally unhappy because the patient is a walking testimonial to what might appear to be the physician's incompetence. The complication of urinary incontinence is happily an infrequent one but probably occurs in about 1 percent of patients undergoing surgery for BPH.

There are two mechanisms that control urinary continence, and each plays a specific role in maintaining a man in a continent and dry state. One is the musculature that surrounds much of the prostate gland, and is outside of the true capsule of the prostate. It serves to maintain the tone of the prostatic urethra and bladder neck and to keep them in a relatively closed position except when a man is voiding. Severe damage to this musculature can lead to profound and total incontinence. The other mechanism for continence is the external urethral sphincter. Damage to this muscle can lead to a stress type of incontinence, which means that there may be an involuntary loss of urine when there is increased pressure within the abdomen that squeezes down on the bladder. Such pressure can occur with sneezing, coughing, physical exertion, etc. Damage to either of these continence mechanisms can occur during the course of the surgery although it may not be recognized at the time. There are very definite landmarks to guide the urologist during the surgical procedure, and whenever surgeon-inflicted damage occurs to the musculature surrounding the prostate gland or to the muscle of the external urethral sphincter, incontinence to a greater or lesser degree may occur. Sometimes, vision may be obscured during the course of a transurethral operation because of heavy bleeding and at other times the problem may result from a relative lack of experience on the part of the urologist. But the fact remains that incontinence will still occasionally be a complication in the hands of even the best and most skilled urologists. The extent of the damage to either continence mechanism will determine the severity of the incontinence; it can vary from a complete and total inability to hold *any* urine in the bladder to a minor and relatively mild loss of urine with severe straining or heavy physical exercise.

When incontinence, of whatever degree, does occur it is not necessarily irreversible or permanent. There are both medical and surgical means of combating this extremely distressing problem. When the urine leakage is due to damage of the musculature surrounding the prostate gland and the prostatic urethra, the undamaged muscle that remains behind can often be stimulated to contract by various drugs and can actually be made to come fairly close to functioning as it did before the injury. The success or failure of this type of therapy will depend upon the extent of damage to the muscles involved, and how well the remaining muscles can be made to function. Drugs such as Ephedrine, for example, act on the remaining musculature that surrounds the prostate gland to make it contract, thereby decreasing the inside measurement of the prostatic urethra and promoting continence. Sometimes this medical regime is combined with drug therapy that acts on the bladder to relax it and to minimize its ability to contract. This can further help the storage of urine in the bladder, and discourage urine leakage to the outside. When the drug therapy is not successful, surgical remedies may well be, but I feel these should not be considered for a minimum of six months, and preferably a year, after surgery so as to be quite certain that continence will not return without surgery.

The last several years have witnessed absolutely remarkable innovations in the development of artificial urinary sphincters, which are usually placed around the urethra just beyond the external urethral sphincter (Fig. 8–1). These sphincters look and function like miniature blood pressure cuffs that surround the urethra and totally occlude it when inflated. The sphincters are kept in the inflated state to prevent urinary leakage. When the patient feels that his bladder is filling he presses a button which is concealed in a pump mechanism buried in the upper part of his scrotum. This deflates the cuff and allows urine to flow freely. The cuff then automatically reinflates about sixty seconds later following bladder emptying. These sphincters are certainly not a panacea for all patients, but they are a gigantic step forward in solving this extremely unfortunate problem. Probably somewhere between 75 and 90 percent of patients in whom these prosthetic devices have been implanted are able to achieve a very satisfactory degree of continence.

Post-TURP Scarring (Stricture) of the Urethra. This is another complication of transurethral surgery, one that is almost totally avoidable. The stricture of the urethra is a scar that can be anywhere in the urethra between the bladder neck and the opening on the end of the penis; but it is most often found in that part of the urethra where the underside of the penis joins the scrotal skin. It is also found commonly just inside the

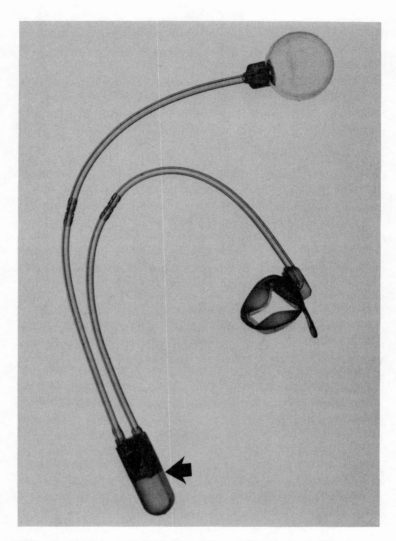

Figure 8–1   *An artificial urinary sphincter. The circular cuff in the center is placed around the urethra just adjacent to the external urethral sphincter. The large, clear reservoir (top) is placed underneath the muscles of the lower abdomen, and the pump mechanism (arrow) is placed in the scrotum. The cuff is kept in the inflated position; when a patient has to urinate he squeezes a button on the pump which allows fluid to go from the cuff back into the reservoir, thereby deflating the cuff and allowing urine to flow out of the bladder. Thirty seconds after the cuff is deflated, and the patient has finished voiding, the cuff automatically reinflates.*

opening on the end of the penis. This stricture or narrowing within the urethra decreases the size of the channel through which the urine flows; so a patient with a significant post-TURP stricture will often have an obstruction to the flow of urine that is as bad or worse than the problem he had that led to the prostate surgery in the first place.

A post-TURP stricture results from trauma to the urethra that may result during the course of a TURP when a patient's urethra is too small for the size of the surgical instrument (the resectoscope) introduced into it. A rough estimate of the frequency of post-TURP strictures is about 10 to 15 percent, although not all of the patients that have these strictures will have any voiding symptoms. They may simply have a urethral channel that is somewhat smaller postoperatively than it was preoperatively. However, the incidence of post-TURP strictures can be reduced to well under 1 percent by measuring the inside of the urethra immediately prior to the insertion of the resectoscope. This is done with a special and very simple instrument. If the inside measurement of the urethra is smaller than a specific size that will vary according to the size of the resectoscope being used, the urethra must be enlarged surgically. This is easily done with another simple instrument that cuts the urethra in its narrowed places so that it will not be too small for the resectoscope. After the surgical procedure has been completed, the part of the urethra that had been cut gradually heals and returns to its normal preoperative size.

If a patient does suffer voiding difficulty from a post-TURP stricture, it can sometimes be treated adequately with periodic stretching of the urethra. But sometimes the strictured area must be cut surgically and allowed to heal around a large-size catheter which ideally will permit the return of the urethra to its preoperative size. Occasionally, a more extensive plastic surgical operation on the urethra must be done to repair the strictured area.

When one of the open types of surgical operation for BPH has been done a postoperative stricture may result at the spot where the urethra was divided. This is a particular risk if the division of the urethra, which is done as virtually the last step

before the obstructing BPH tissue is actually removed, is not
done cleanly and sharply.

Bladder Neck Contracture. This is an infrequent (about 1 percent) but extremely troublesome complication that can occur
when very small enlargements of the prostate—that perhaps
do not really warrant surgery—are in fact surgically removed.
These very small prostatic enlargements are located entirely
within the prostatic urethra and do not extend upwards towards
the bladder, so they do not overlie the bladder neck. When
operating on these very small prostatic enlargements, therefore, the urologist may find himself cutting away normal
bladder neck instead of BPH tissue. The injured bladder neck
then tends to heal by scar formation. This will often leave a
patient with an extraordinarily small opening in the bladder
neck through which the urine must flow. This opening can be
as small as a pinhead and will cause the patient to have a
recurrence of the symptoms for which he had his prostatic
surgery in the first place. The new symptoms, however, are
often more severe and pronounced than were those of the
prostatic enlargement (BPH). The problem is treated by cutting the bladder neck and is done through a cystoscope, usually with the patient asleep. This cutting may need to be done
again because the narrowing of the bladder neck tends to recur.
Happily, a bladder neck narrowing is a very infrequent complication of prostatic surgery and is much more easily prevented than treated.

Sexual Problems. The ability to achieve an erection that is satisfactory for sexual intercourse is obviously very important.
So important, in fact, that many men often delay seeking
treatment for medical problems because they fear that the
treatment itself may cause them to become impotent. This is
often the case with BPH because the myth persists that a man's
sex life is over when he has prostate surgery for the relief of
BPH. Men, therefore, often delay such surgery to the great
detriment of their health and well-being. Moreover, they often
enter into the surgery convinced that their sexually active days
are behind them. In fact, nothing could be further from the

truth, but it is this preconceived notion that is one of the factors making it so very difficult to assess accurately the true incidence of postoperative loss of erectile function. If such a loss occurs, it may be due to damage from the surgery itself, but it may also be psychogenic because a patient *anticipated* that it would happen.

Another major factor obscuring the cause-and-effect relationship of surgery for BPH and postoperative impotence is the effect that *any* surgery can have on erectile function, an effect probably due to a combination of psychogenic and organic stimuli from the general bodily insult that results from any surgical procedure, and not to specific damage to any structures that affect potency. Studies comparing the incidence of preoperative and postoperative impotence among patients undergoing prostatectomy and patients undergoing general surgical procedures on the abdomen (but not including any surgery on the prostate) show that the incidence of impotence is extraordinarily similar before and after surgery regardless of whether the surgery was done on the prostate gland or on some other abdominal structure. The incidence of preoperative and postoperative impotence appears to be directly age-related; the older the age group the greater the incidence of preoperative and postoperative impotence. Since the age and numbers of patients undergoing prostatic surgery for the relief of BPH is probably greater than the age of patients having other surgical procedures, it is certainly possible, although unproven, that any increase in impotence following prostate surgery as compared to the impotence following other surgical procedures is purely age-related.

Yet another obscuring factor that is even more important is the extreme difficulty in accurately assessing a man's erectile function prior to and following prostate surgery. In my experience, a man will often exaggerate his abilities preoperatively and then say that his poor function postoperatively is a result of surgery when, in fact, his sexual function was as poor before surgery as it was afterwards. Unless meticulous studies using standardized criteria, and including interviews with the patients' spouses, are included in the scientific data obtained about the results of prostate surgery on erectile function, the answers to many specific questions will remain obscure. In reviewing a great deal of literature on the subject, there is a range of 5 to 34 percent of men who claim to have been functioning well sexually prior to surgery but then were unable to have adequate erections afterwards. In my experience, the figure is much nearer to 5 percent, but I always spend a great deal of time telling a patient prior to surgery that his sexual abilities preoperatively will be pretty much the same postoperatively. I also tell a patient that he should not anticipate any diminishing in his ability to perform intercourse as a result of the surgery. There is certainly no physiologic reason that a properly done operation on the prostate for BPH should result in any impairment of erectile function, although it clearly does on occasion. Whether these occasions represent psychogenic influences or whether, in some extraordinary manner, damage occurs to one or both of the nerve bundles which control erections, is problematic. There is one such nerve bundle on each side of the prostate gland but they are *outside* of the true capsule. There is, therefore, no reason whatever for a surgical instrument to come in contact with one of these nerve bundles in the usual and ordinary type of prostate surgery for BPH.

However, in the last analysis, if a patient does experience erectile inadequacy following surgery, he could and should be treated exactly as a patient with a similar problem who has not had prostatic surgery. The means of treatment include a diagnostic workup to try and determine the cause of the erectile dysfunction and, indeed, establishing with certainty that there is an organic and not a psychologic cause for the problem. This is usually done by using a machine to monitor whether or not erections occur during sleep, since erections normally occur several times a night during sleep and this continues with psychogenic but not true organic impotence.

Treatment of impotence, whether organic or psychologic, can be done using various drugs (principally papaverine, and / or Prostaglandin E which brings an increased blood supply to the penis) that are injected directly into the penis or, alternatively, by means of implanting one of the several different available types of prosthesis into the penis. The drug injections are initially done by the urologist but the patient is then taught how to do them himself. If followed by sexual foreplay, they will result in a firm erection that lasts for one or two hours or longer. The patient is instructed to use the injections a maximum of eight times per month. Most patients using this new method feel that it does indeed result in excellent erections. Some patients maintain themselves on this regime for several years, although there are some risks to the procedure itself and some patients ultimately tire of it. I must point out that this form of therapy, although used extensively by many urologists, does not, as of 1993, have FDA (Food and Drug Administration) approval.

A very exciting new means of producing erection that is still in the research stage is the instillation, by the patient, directly into his urethra of a small pellet that is absorbed through the lining of the urethra and results in an erection.

Still another form of therapy is the use of a vacuum device. This is a cylinder into which the flaccid penis is placed. The air is then manually pumped out of the cylinder and this results in an erection which may be maintained for up to a half hour by means of a constricting band that is placed around the base of the penis just before the cylinder is removed from the penis.

An alternative therapy is the implantation of one of the various kinds of penile prostheses, which goes into the spongy bodies of the penis and stiffens them to allow for penetration during intercourse. Although there are many different brands of penile prostheses, the two fundamental types are the semirigid and the inflatable (Figs. 8–2, 8–3). Each of these has several advantages and disadvantages and the ultimate decision as to which type to use is properly a decision made jointly by the patient and his urologist.

Retrograde Ejaculation. Retrograde ejaculation is an occurrence affecting between one-half and two-thirds of patients undergoing prostatic surgery for BPH. When it does occur following surgery the result is a "dry ejaculate." This is because at the time of ejaculation the semen follows the path of least resistance, which is backwards into the bladder. During the course of prostate surgery the bladder neck is often enlarged

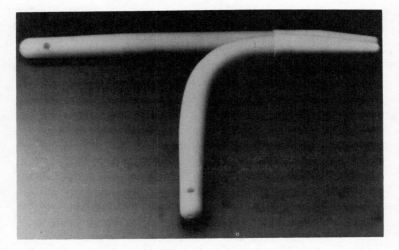

Figure 8–2   *Semi-rigid (malleable) penile prosthesis. This type of prosthesis has virtually no working parts that can break or malfunction, but the penis is always rigid. A patient is, however, able to bend his penis so that it points downward along the inner part of his thigh and does not interfere with usual daily activity. When intercourse is desired, the penis can be bent upward so that it sticks straight out. To illustrate this, the photograph shows one of the two paired prostheses bent in the downward position, and the other in the upward or fully erect position.*

and is therefore not able to close completely (as it normally does) during orgasm and ejaculation. When the bladder neck does not close, the semen, which enters the prostatic portion of the urethra from the ejaculatory ducts, flows in a backward direction through the incompletely closed bladder neck and into the bladder. This should be of no consequence whatever to the patient since the feeling at the time of orgasm and ejaculation is unchanged from what it was prior to surgery. But the retrograde ejaculation would make the likelihood of fathering a child extremely slight. As a general rule, almost all patients undergoing surgery for BPH are beyond the age where fatherhood is of interest to them, but it is absolutely amazing to me that many patients are extremely annoyed, and even angry, when they find that they have retrograde ejaculation unless they have been forewarned of this. In my experience, as long as a patient has been advised of the possibility of retrograde ejaculation occurring, it is accepted with equanimity if it does indeed occur.

In the event that retrograde ejaculation does occur in an individual who is intent on fathering more children, there are techniques that are readily available to isolate the semen from the urine which is voided immediately after ejaculation. These techniques are neither difficult nor exotic, and the semen which is recovered can be injected into the vagina, in close proximity to the cervix, in the same manner that artificial insemination is done.

Epididymitis. This is a complication of prostate surgery that may occur while a patient is in the hospital, but it usually occurs two to six weeks following surgery when the patient is well on his way to recovery at home. It is a condition in which there

Figure 8–3 Inflatable prostheses. *This type of prosthesis allows for an increase in girth as well as rigidity of the penis when the device is inflated; it also allows for a normal flaccid state of the penis when the device is deflated. (Illustrations courtesy of American Medical Systems, Minnetonka, Minnesota)*

A. The self-contained penile prosthesis which consists of paired cylinders totally contained within the penis. By pumping behind the head of the penis, fluid is transferred from the rear portion of the device to the part of the device contained within the shaft of the penis. The cylinder thus becomes enlarged and produces a firm penis. When an erection is no longer desired, the fluid is returned to the rear reservoir through a side channel by pressing the release valve located behind the pump.

B. The most frequently used inflatable device in which the pump (arrow) which is placed within the scrotum is squeezed thereby transferring fluid from the fluid reservoir (top of photo) into the paired cylinders, making the penis increase in girth and rigidity. When the erection is no longer desired, a release valve on the pump permits the transfer of fluid from the cylinders back into the reservoir.

C. An artist's drawing showing where the various parts of the inflatable device illustrated in (b) are placed anatomically. Top: the penis is flaccid and the prosthesis is deflated. Bottom: the penis is erect and the prosthesis is inflated. Note the increase in the size of the cylinders when the penis is rigid and the corresponding decrease in the size of the reservoir since much of the fluid has been transferred from the reservoir to the cylinders.

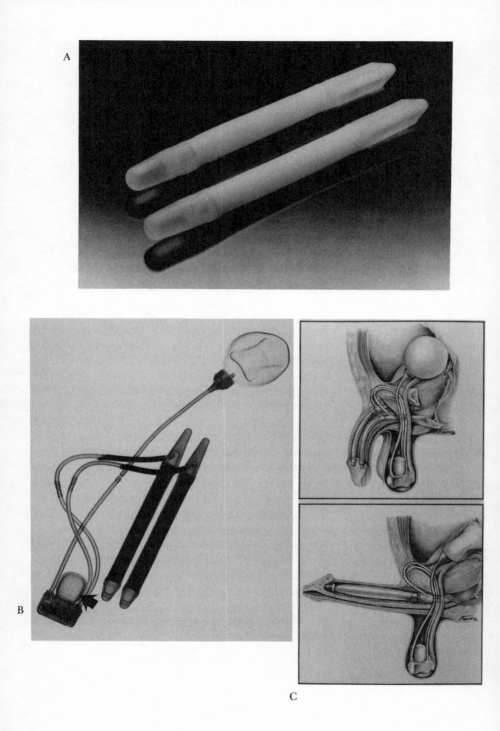

is a pronounced inflammation and enlargement of the epididymis (Chapter 1) accompanied by considerable pain and tenderness. The inflammatory process not infrequently also involves the adjacent testis producing a large, hard, extremely tender mass within the scrotum that can be as large as a plum or even a small peach. Epididymitis is an uncommon complication of prostate surgery that probably occurs in 2 to 3 percent of patients, and it is most likely to occur if a patient had infected urine preoperatively or a prior history of epididymitis. Until ten or twenty years ago most patients undergoing prostate surgery had a bilateral vasectomy done immediately prior to the prostate surgery. Although a bilateral vasectomy is a very common operation for the purposes of voluntary sterilization, when it is done immediately prior to surgery for BPH it is done specifically to prevent any bacteria that may be present in the bladder or the prostate or the prostatic urethra from traveling down the vas deferens and into the epididymis. Most urologists no longer routinely do a vasectomy before prostate surgery, but the incidence of postoperative epididymitis remains very minimal. When it does occur, the acute discomfort usually goes away in one to two weeks but the swelling can take up to ten to twelve weeks to resolve completely. Treatment is with antibiotics, pain medications, and rest. A scrotal support is also helpful.

Persistent Bacteriuria. Following prostatic surgery for benign disease it takes two to four months before the prostatic urethra has formed its new lining. This is because during the course of the surgery the prostatic urethra is removed along with the obstructing prostate tissue. The lining of the bladder subsequently extends downwards into the prostatic urethra to form a new lining. During this period when the area of the prostatic urethra is healing, there is a constant shedding of white blood cells (pus cells). This is a normal part of the healing process. It does not mean that infection is necessarily present. So, even though there are many white blood cells in the urine of patients recovering from prostate surgery, it does not necessarily mean that any bacterial infection is present in the urine. Indeed, if bacteria *are* present in the urine of patients who are recovering from prostatic surgery it is abnormal and should be treated. The usual treatment consists of several days of an antibiotic to which the bacteria are susceptible. If it is not possible to sterilize the urine by this means or if the infection recurs after successful treatment, then a thorough investigation is necessary to look for those causes of infection that may have been overlooked and that generally require further treatment. Such things as incomplete bladder emptying, which may or may not be due to incomplete removal of the obstructing BPH tissue, bladder diverticulae (outpouchings usually caused by BPH, see Chapter 4) that do not empty, or even obstruction to the drainage of a kidney that has bacteria in it can all result in recurrent infection following prostatic surgery. When the reason for the infection has been found, treatment can usually correct it. Some urologists prefer to keep patients on antibiotics for several weeks following surgery whereas others prefer to treat infections if they occur. While I tend to agree with the latter, it may certainly be said that there is no right or wrong in this issue, and a physician will generally follow the course that he or she has found to be most successful in the past.

Surgery for Cancer of
the Prostate

Transurethral Surgery

Complications that can occur when a transurethral prostatic operation is done for a patient with prostatic cancer who has symptoms of bladder outlet obstruction due to a coexisting BPH are the same as those that can occur when the operation is done for BPH. This is particularly true when the obstructing tissue is predominantly benign. This is a common occurrence, since you will recall that cancer of the prostate and BPH both occur in the same age group.

However, if the transurethral surgery is done to relieve the obstructive symptoms caused by an advanced cancer of the prostate, then the complications of the surgery are much more severe. This is because when the entire prostate is pretty well replaced by cancerous tissue the prostatic urethra becomes more of a rigid tube and not at all pliable. Since one of the mechanisms for continence depends upon the pliability of the prostatic urethra, so that it can virtually close off this channel at times, it is obvious that if the cancer turns the prostatic urethra into a rigid structure continence could become a real problem. Incontinence of urine does, in fact, occur in about 5 percent of patients who have TURs to relieve the obstructive symptoms of advanced prostatic cancer. Bleeding following a TUR for advanced cancer of the prostate can also be a formidable problem because there are certain substances in the cancerous tissue itself that tend to promote bleeding and prevent the usual process of blood coagulation through which bleeding usually stops. Finally, it should be recalled that a TUR of the prostate with advanced and extensive malignancy in it must be looked on as a purely palliative procedure to alleviate voiding difficulties and is certainly not curative of the cancer.

Radical (Total) Prostatectomy

Incontinence. When a radical prostatectomy is done in an attempt to achieve a cure or a long-term survival in a patient with prostate cancer, the entire prostate gland is removed along with the prostatic urethra. A gap in the continuity of the urethra is obviously created. It is bridged by bringing the bladder neck down to the remaining portion of the urethra at the level of the external urethral spincter. The bladder neck is then stitched to that remaining urethra. Obviously, therefore, when a portion of urethra several centimeters long is removed there is always going to be a chance of urinary incontinence even if the reconstruction of the urethra is perfectly done. In fact, between two and 5 percent of patients undergoing radical prostatectomy do suffer from a severe, or even total, incontinence. An even higher percentage may have involuntary loss of urine for a short time following surgery or may have a mild degree of incontinence (such as stress incontinence) for a prolonged period of time. When an involuntary loss of urine persists beyond the period of hospitalization, various medications may be used in an attempt to minimize the incontinence. These are the same medications that are used for incontinence following prostate surgery for BPH (see Chapter 4).

Another technique to treat incontinence, and the one I try to teach to my patients as soon as the catheter is removed following a radical prostatectomy, is the so-called Kegel exercise. This is an exercise in which the patient himself embarks on a regular schedule to add tone and strength to the muscles that control continence. There are actually two groups of muscles that are used, the first of which is around the rectum and the second around the base of the penis. The first is the muscle you tighten when you want to suddenly stop the flow of urine while you are voiding. The second of these muscle groups is the one you would use when you think you are through voiding and want to expel the last few drops or the last "squirt" of urine. These two groups of muscles should be contracted sequentially, starting with the one you would use to stop the flow of urine while voiding and then, while keeping that muscle contracted, additionally contracting the muscle that you would use to get out the last "squirt" of urine at the end of voiding. You should contract and hold in a contracted state—as tightly as you can—both of these sets of muscles for 10 seconds and do this at least half a dozen times a day with at least a few minutes rest between contractions. You should also make a conscious effort to contract these muscles before lifting or straining or doing anything that might place an increased pressure on your bladder and result in an involuntary urine loss.

In the course of the healing process after a radical prostatectomy, improvement in the regaining of continence can be anticipated for up to a year following surgery. If the incontinence of urine is still sufficient to cause distress to a patient beyond that point, an artificial sphincter can be surgically implanted as already described for the incontinence that can result from surgery for benign prostatic disease. These artificial sphincters, while certainly not totally effective in all patients, do provide significant improvement and sometimes total cure in a majority of patients in whom they are implanted.

Contracture of the Bladder Neck. Contracture of the bladder neck at the area where it is stitched to the remaining portion of the urethra is a not infrequent complication of radical prostate surgery. It occurs within the first three months after the operation. Typically, the patient will note that his urinary stream diminishes in force and caliber sharply, and he has difficulty voiding. These are the same symptoms as those of a bladder neck contracture following prostatic surgery for BPH. Even though the cause of the contracture is different, the treatment remains the same. A knife cut in the contracted bladder neck that is done transurethrally, or even better the passage of a dilating instrument through the urethra past the contracted area, may work well. It is uncommon for this particular complication of bladder neck contracture to persist or to recur once it has been treated.

Erectile Dysfunction. Erectile dysfunction used to occur in the great majority of patients undergoing radical prostatectomy. But in the last several years a modification of the radical surgical procedure has been developed that spares the nerves which control erection. These nerves run very close to the prostate gland in small bundles on either side of the prostate. When the nerve-sparing operative procedure is done successfully, erectile function remains fairly good in many patients. There are urologists, however, who remain concerned that by sparing the nerves controlling erection the efficacy of a good cancer operation may be compromised and that some cancer cells may be left behind in the patient. This is because in order to spare the nerves it is necessary to "shave" the margins of the prostate gland quite closely, so that if the cancer goes right up to the true capsule of the prostate and perhaps through it, there is a possibility of leaving some cancer cells behind in the patient. Whether or not the nerve-sparing operation will ultimately be used only in patients with a very small focus of cancer that is well removed from the side margins of the prostate gland remains to be seen, but at this time the operation has not been in use long enough to say with certainty whether it compromises the success of an operation which is designed to rid the patient of his cancer and to cure him. I must also point out that sometimes potency can be maintained by preserving the nerve on only one side; but there are urologists who nevertheless feel that the preferred operation for cancer is to take the widest margins possible on *both* sides of the prostate, thereby destroying both nerves.

If no attempt is made to spare the nerves then the operation as it is now carried out will result in erectile dysfunction and impotence for most patients following surgery. If this impotence does occur it is treated in the same manner as erectile dysfunction that occurs following surgery for benign prostatic disease. In the case of the radical prostatectomy, however, the intrapenile injections of prostaglandin or papaverine (or often a combination of the two and sometimes with the addition of regitine as well) are not always as successful as they are when erectile dysfunction occurs following surgery for benign disease. This is because some of the blood supply to the penis (in addition to the nerves) may be destroyed during radical prostatectomy. Therefore, a drug designed to increase the blood flow through existing blood vessels simply will not work. The success of the intrapenile injections following radical prostatectomy seems to be related in large part to the age of the patient. Not surprisingly, the younger the patient, the better the chance of success; this is because younger patients will have better blood vessels (throughout the body and not just leading into the penis). Therefore, assuming minimal damage to the blood vessels supplying the penis during surgery, a younger patient will anticipate a better result from the injections. If the injections do not work or if the patient is not interested in having this kind of treatment, then the intrapenile prostheses are indeed successful and an excellent form of therapy. The use of these prosthetic devices following radical prostatectomy is the same as that following the surgery for benign disease.

The latest, still experimental but extremely exciting advance in the treatment of postsurgical impotence (as well as other forms of impotence) is the administration of prostaglandin and papaverine in pellet form directly into the urethra by means of a small eye-dropper-like device. This ingenious method of delivering the medication so that it is absorbed into the spongy bodies of the penis may well replace the intrapenile injections in the future. At present, however, the method is under clinical investigation at various university sites around the country. Early results are extremely promising, but general availability of this form of medication will very likely not receive FDA approval until 1995 or later.

The impotence often associated with prostate cancer, and indeed the prostate cancer itself, are often understandably the cause of great concern and anxiety to many men. For some, the presence of a support group of men who have been through a similar experience may be most helpful. There are several support groups in this country for men with prostate cancer; perhaps the largest and best known is an organization known as "US TOO." This organization has about 170 local chapters in North America (most of them in the United States) and you can find the one nearest to you by calling 1-800-828-7866. The address of "US TOO" headquarters is 300 West Pratt Street, Suite 401, Baltimore Maryland 21201.

Some General Comments

The kind of complications discussed in this chapter that can occur when prostate surgery is done either for benign prostatic hyperplasia or for cancer are not common but they certainly can and do occur. In the present-day atmosphere it is generally accepted that informed patients who fully understand their surgery often do better postoperatively and have better results. Moreover, a patient is *entitled* to know and understand a contemplated surgical procedure. For these reasons, the concept of informed consent is one that has gained widespread acceptance both in medical and in legal circles. This simply means that when a patient gives his consent for an operation he has been informed about what the operation is, what the risks are, and what the potential complications are. It is sometimes a difficult balancing act for a urologist to determine just exactly how much detail a patient might want to know or should know about the risks and complications of surgery. Unquestionably, a presentation covering every con-

ceivably bad thing that might happen to a patient and covering it in lurid detail might well scare the patient away from
needed surgery or might well send the patient into a surgical
procedure with enormous apprehension about possible complications. On the other hand, it is unquestionably a patient's
right to know about the things that might go wrong with an
operation so that he can have the opportunity to refuse the
surgery if he wants to.

When I am discussing the subject of risks and complications with my patient I will always answer in an honest and
forthright way any direct questions that they ask me and I will
be as frank with my patients as I would want my own doctor
to be with me. However, I do not think it particularly wise or
helpful to a patient to scare him before an operation by bringing up things that are most unlikely to happen, particularly
when these are things that the patient has never even considered. Most of my patients want to know what the risks are
in terms of mortality and I tell them this truthfully, to my best
knowledge. Most of the patients also want to know about the
possibility of incontinence and I answer this as truthfully as I
can. Some of my patients ask about the sexual activity they
might anticipate following surgery and I always explain this
in great detail; in fact, this is one subject that I will bring up
if a patient fails to ask anything about it.

Radiation Therapy

Occasionally, in selected cases, radiation therapy is used
for the treatment of prostatic cancer. Not infrequently the
complications of this form of treatment can be every bit as
significant to the patient as the complications of radical surgery.

About 50 percent of patients undergoing radiation therapy for prostatic cancer will suffer from erectile dysfunction
and impotence as a result of the therapy, and it is *not* psychogenic impotence. The precise mechanism responsible for this
loss of erectile function is not well understood, but it is probably related to the effect of the radiation on the blood vessels

supplying the spongy parts within the penis. Treatment of this condition often requires one of the penis implants as described above, although the penile injections and / or the vacuum device will certainly help some patients.

Unfortunately a minority, albeit a significant minority, of patients will occasionally suffer from radiation effects to the rectum and to the bladder. It is often said by radiation therapists that when this type of treatment is properly delivered by a skilled individual, the radiation effects on the rectum or bladder are virtually nil. In my experience, however, a minority—perhaps up to 10 percent—of patients undergoing radiation therapy do end up with long-term symptoms of bladder, and possibly even rectal, distress. The rectal symptoms occur less often than those affecting the bladder and are generally those producing frequency of bowel movements or diarrhea. The bladder symptoms are those of urinary frequency that not uncommonly results in the need to void every ten to forty minutes day and night and in bleeding from the bladder. When these unpleasant symptoms occur there is relatively little that can be done to relieve them other than to hope that eventually the symptoms will go away. Unfortunately, these symptoms—particularly those affecting the bladder—tend to last for a long time.

9

Final Thoughts on Lots of Subjects

In the six years that have elapsed since I first wrote this book, a great deal of progress has continued to advance and enhance the diagnosis and treatment of prostatic diseases. Some methods and techniques that I described then as being new are now no longer new, and there is much additional information about which I can tell you. Moreover, there has been a good deal of new knowledge generated in the inevitable forward progress in the art and science of urology. It is for these reasons, and to ensure that this book is as up to date as possible, that I have written this chapter for the current edition of *The Prostate Book*. Finally, numerous individuals who read the original book have been kind enough to write to me or to telephone with very specific questions and problems, some of which were obviously not adequately addressed in the earlier book. Some of these people were concerned about sexual problems that resulted following surgery for benign prostatic hyperplasia (BPH); others simply wanted to talk about a variety of their own problems; still others wanted to know about newer treatments not covered at all in the original book. In this chapter I will try to bring your knowledge of the prostate and many of its problems to the current level of knowledge, and I will also address many of the queries that I have received in the past two years. I will follow the original chapter headings as much as possible in doing this.

Chapter 2: How the Doctor Diagnoses Your Problem

Prostate specific antigen (pages 31–33), or PSA, is now universally regarded as the preferred blood test that is used in association with cancer of the prostate. You should not, however, look upon it as a test by which your doctor can say with certainty that you do or do not have cancer of the prostate. In other words, it should not be considered as being specific for prostate cancer. It is a very sensitive test, and is thought by many clinicians to be a good screening test for very early disease recognition. The problem with such early detection is that we don't know if or how it will affect the death rate from prostate cancer. Whether your prostate gland feels normal or abnormal to your doctor when he performs a digital rectal examination on you (see page 91), a normal PSA blood level will still not be able to say definitively that you do *not* have prostate cancer. On the other hand, if your prostate gland feels perfectly normal, and if the PSA is elevated (the normal range is 0–4.0 ng / ml), it *may* indicate the presence of prostate cancer. If your prostate gland feels abnormal and the PSA is elevated above the normal range, this also *may* indicate the presence of prostate cancer.

Although the PSA blood test does indeed represent a truly remarkable advance that urologists employ almost daily as a helpful tool in the diagnosis and management of patients with prostate cancer, it must be remembered that PSA is made by the cells of the prostate, both benign cells and malignant cells, and its level can be elevated above the normal range if you have a particularly large, but benign, prostate gland. It has also been found to be elevated above the normal range if there is pronounced inflammation (prostatitis) present (see Chapter 3) or if a prostatic infarction is present (a harmless and uncommon condition, often producing no symptoms, in which there is a sudden blockage of the blood supply to a portion of the prostate gland). These conditions—BPH, prostatitis, and infarction—may raise the PSA level to two or three times the normal upper limit and occasionally even beyond this point. As a general rule, however, a PSA level that is higher than 10–15 ng / ml, in the absence of BPH, prostatitis, or infarction, is highly suspicious for prostate cancer. A PSA value that is well within the limits of normal, I must repeat, very definitely does *not* eliminate the diagnosis of prostate cancer, and this is particularly true in the presence of a palpable abnormality of the prostate on digital rectal examination.

Malignant prostate cells can make up to ten times as much PSA per gram of tissue as can benign prostate cells; this is one reason for the elevation of PSA that is seen with prostate cancer. For this same reason the PSA level will also be dependent upon the volume (the amount) of the cancer just as it will vary directly with the volume of BPH. Since malignant cells make more PSA than benign cells, however, the PSA level will be higher for a given volume of cancer cells as compared with the same volume of BPH.

As I have said more than once, the PSA value does not by itself have the ability to indicate whether you definitely do or do not have prostate cancer, although it is certainly fair to say that the higher the PSA value, the greater the likelihood that prostate cancer is present. The problem is that benign enlargement of the prostate (BPH) will also cause the PSA level to rise, although, gram for gram, malignant (cancer) prostate tissue will result in a higher PSA value than will benign prostate tissue. Infection or inflammation within the prostate will also, as noted above, cause a rise in the PSA value. In an effort to try to predict which elevated PSA values are more likely to be cancer and which are not, many urologists con-

sider the PSA density to be helpful (but certainly not definitive). This PSA density concept is based on the fact that, per
gram of prostate tissue, cancer cells will make more PSA than
will benign tissue. When an ultrasound examination of the
prostate is done (usually in conjunction with the prostate
biopsy), it is possible to determine the size (in cubic centimeters) and the weight (in grams) of the entire prostate. The
PSA density is then calculated by dividing the PSA value by
the weight of the prostate in grams. If the number resulting
from this determination (the PSA density) is 0.15 or less the
odds are against the presence of cancer. If the resulting PSA
density is 0.2 or higher the odds of cancer being present in
the prostate are increased. The concept of PSA density is an
interesting one; it is also logical because it is based on the truism
that the higher the PSA value per weight of the prostate gland
the greater the chances of cancer. This is because, as already
said, malignant prostate tissue makes ten times as much PSA
as does benign prostate tissue. However, I must again emphasize that neither the PSA value nor the PSA density is able, by
itself, to say with any degree of certainty that prostate cancer
is present. The definitive diagnosis must be made by biopsy.

In my own practice, I generally use the following rule of
thumb as regards PSA levels. If my patient has a prostate gland
that feels normal on digital rectal examination and if his PSA
level is under 4 ng / ml, I will do nothing except recommend
an annual digital rectal examination and PSA blood level. If
the prostate gland feels abnormal (suspicious for the possibility of prostate cancer), then I will do a biopsy of the prostate
gland (see pages 59–68) regardless of whether the PSA level
is normal or elevated. If the digital rectal examination of the
prostate is normal, and the PSA is elevated very minimally
above 4 ng / ml, then I may just repeat the PSA in three months
to see if it is rising. Usually, however, I will do an ultrasound
of the prostate (see pages 40–42), to look for hypoechoic areas
that may represent carcinoma. Such areas, I feel, should then
be biopsied under ultrasound guidance. To summarize this
last point, in evaluating patients who have a normal prostate
by palpation and an elevated PSA level (above 4 ng / ml), please

keep in mind that there is a strong likelihood that this PSA elevation is due to a benign condition such as enlargement of the prostate, previous or present inflammation of the prostate, and / or infarction of the prostate. It is, however, my firm belief that these patients should, as a general rule, have a prostatic ultrasound and a biopsy of any areas that are seen to be hypoechoic and that suggest the possibility of prostate cancer. If no hypoechoic areas are seen, I believe that six random biopsies from different areas of the prostate are indicated.

The foregoing is my general rule of thumb in matters concerning PSA levels in my patients. However, as noted much earlier in this book, PSA is made by both benign and malignant prostate cells and therefore its numerical value will vary with the size or volume of the prostate (although it still remains true that gram for gram malignant prostate tissue will make about ten times as much PSA as will benign prostate tissue). Because of this dependency upon the size of the prostate, and because older men tend to have larger prostates than younger men, recent studies have shown that the upper limit of 4ng / ml of PSA may not accurately reflect the amounts of PSA normally put out by the larger prostates of older men. Also, since younger men tend to have smaller prostates, the upper limit of 4ng / ml of PSA may be too high in younger men. Many urologists now believe that in men up to age 45, 2.5 ng / ml of PSA is a more reasonable upper limit for normal values; in men 60–69, 4.5 ng / ml of PSA is a reasonable upper limit of normal; and in men 70–79, 6.5 ng / ml is within the acceptable limits for a normal value. My previous comments about the need for a prostate biopsy of a prostate that feels abnormal regardless of the PSA value remain unchanged.

PSA levels may also be dependent upon the *ploidy* (see below) of the cancer (assuming that cancer is indeed present) and in some cases aneuploid and tetraploid cancers may produce higher PSA levels than will the more common diploid cancers. "Ploidy" is the abbreviation for "nuclear DNA ploidy pattern" and this is the pattern of the total DNA content of the nuclei of a given sample of tissue as plotted on a graph that is known as a histogram. DNA stands for deoxyribonucleic acid, which is a complex protein found in all cells. The process by which these graphs or histograms are plotted based on the DNA content in the nuclei of the cancerous tissue cells is called "flow cytometry," a highly sophisticated and technically complex procedure that is based on the fact that most tumor cells have abnormal amounts of DNA. I will have more to say on the ploidy pattern of prostate cancers below when I discuss the surgical treatment and survival statistics of prostate cancer. One thing you should know at this time, however, is that the diploid pattern of DNA that is found in most prostate cancers is the same as the DNA pattern found in benign prostate tissue, and so the presence of a diploid pattern on the DNA histogram cannot be used to determine the presence or absence of malignancy. A biopsy with a microscopic examination of the overall appearance and of the specific cells in the biopsy specimen (see pages 56–68) remains the way that malignancy (cancer) is diagnosed.

Ultrasound of the prostate (see pages 39–41, 66–67) has become infinitely more sophisticated and more commonplace in the past few years because of increasing experience with this diagnostic test and because of increasing excellence in the quality of the ultrasound equipment. Most urologists still feel, and I agree with this, that it should not be used as a screening test to determine if a man does or does not have prostate cancer in those individuals in whom the digital rectal exam is totally normal and the PSA level is also normal. The reason for this is that it is not a cost-efficient study from the patient's point of view, considering the great infrequency with which prostate cancer can be diagnosed by ultrasound when the digital rectal examination and the PSA level are totally normal.

An even greater reason for not using ultrasound as a screening test is the great number of false positives that are encountered. Most prostate cancers appear hypoechoic or less dense on ultrasound than the surrounding tissue (see photograph on page 67), although about one-quarter of the prostate cancers have the same density as the surrounding tissue. It is the hypoechoic areas, therefore, that are the "suspicious" areas and that are the sites for biopsy. As it turns out, however, of every four or five hypoechoic areas that are biopsied, only one will turn out to be cancerous. The many false positives on ultrasound inevitably mean that many needless biopsies would be performed in the patient in whom the digital rectal exam and the PSA level are normal.

Finally, it has yet to be demonstrated that the incidental discovery of small prostate cancers by ultrasound in the presence of a normal digital rectal prostate exam and a normal PSA level will change the anticipated survival rates for those patients. This is not to say that it would or would not change these survival rates; only that it has not been studied and to do this would take a lengthy study of 10 to 20 years.

For all of these reasons, most urologists do not employ ultrasound technology to *screen* for prostate cancer. However, the quantum leap forward in ultrasound use in the past four years in facilitating the diagnosis of prostate cancer has been its use in those patients felt to have a suspicious or an abnormal prostate on digital rectal examination. In these patients the accuracy of biopsy of the palpably suspicious area has been increased greatly by visualizing this area under ultrasound control, thereby making it possible to direct the biopsy needle directly into it. Another role for prostate ultrasound is for the patient with a palpably normal prostate but with an elevated prostate specific antigen (PSA) level, a situation in which the possibility of prostate cancer definitely exists. In this situation, where there is no abnormal or suspicious area of the prostate to locate with ultrasound, any hypoechoic areas that are seen will be biopsied. In either of these situations, the biopsy is most often done with a "gun" that enables biopsies to be taken with such extremely rapid speed that the procedure is almost painless. For these reasons, most urologists presently prefer to perform prostate biopsies with the biopsy "gun" under ultrasound guidance.

Chapter 4: Benign Prostate Hyperplasia (BPH)

On page 114 I said that "there really is no noninvasive or nonsurgical treatment for benign prostatic hyperplasia that is as successful as surgery." I still firmly believe that a transurethral resection of the prostate (TURP) is the "gold standard" for BPH *when it requires treatment,* but in the past four or five years a good deal of effort and study has led to other methods of treatment that have become available and about which you should certainly be aware. There are at least three good reasons for the recent flurry of activity to find acceptable alternative forms of treatment for BPH.

First is the tremendous financial burden upon the American health care system of performing nearly half a million operations annually on the prostate, and the stimulus has been from the federal government (Medicare) as well as other health insurance providers to find less costly methods of treating BPH.

A second reason, in my opinion, is the extraordinary degree of innovation, love of gadgetry, and an ever present desire to find a better way to do things that so characterizes the minds of many urologists. Urology is, after all, a procedure-based specialty and one particularly amenable to high-tech equipment and innovation.

Yet another reason for seeking alternative methods of treating BPH stems from the very surprising results that were published in the late 1980s by a group of researchers who studied, in retrospect, thousands of patients who had undergone TURP. They analyzed this patient data in terms of quality of life and long-term longevity. It is extremely important to note that none of the patients studied was operated on in the United States where the expertise in transurethral surgery is generally conceded to be superior to that in most other countries (the patients studied were in Denmark, England, and Canada). These studies, however, showed that within eight years after having had a TURP, 20 percent of the patients had to have additional surgery on the prostate or on the urethra, and the long-term (within eight years) mortality of patients following TURP was higher than that of a similar group of patients who had undergone "open" prostatic surgery (pages 163–69) in that same time period. The point of this study was not so much to advocate "open" prostatic surgery as to point out that there *might* be something inherently deleterious in the TURP operation.

Recalling that the patients studied did not have their surgery in the United States, it is my feeling that perhaps the great majority of those who required *additional* operative treatment required this because of an incomplete resection of the prostate performed by a surgeon who possibly did not have the skill or the high level of training of his counterpart in this country. Most of the other repeat surgery that was required was on the urethra because of the occurrence of what should usually be a quite preventable stricture of the urethra following TURP (pages 209–12). I truly believe that the rate of similar complications following TURP is far lower when these procedures are done by the splendidly trained urologists in the United States, and this opinion is amply supported in our own urologic literature.

The question of the higher mortality over an eight-year follow-up period after TURP as compared with "open" removal of the benign prostatic tissue is troublesome and one that I believe may well be a reflection of the fact that in this large series of patients done in foreign countries, those patients who were felt to be poorer surgical risks because of heart disease, lung disease, etc., were operated on transurethrally while those patients who were healthier were operated upon via an "open" operation. This is purely conjecture on my part, however, and it is worth noting that the researchers writing this paper did indeed make every effort to see that the patients in the two groups studied (those having TURP surgery and those having "open" prostate surgery) had similar states of health.

This possible link between a TURP and increased mortality is troubling enough that the American Urological Association and the Federal Agency for Health Care Policy and Research have been jointly funding a project to study this question after which it is hoped that a more extensive and long-term study may be carried out if additional funding by the Federal Agency for Health Care Policy and Research becomes available. The purpose of these studies is to determine if in fact there is an increased mortality among those patients undergoing a TURP as compared to patients having "open" prostate surgery and if that mortality is a result of having had the transurethral operation itself. A second, and equally important, part of this study is to compare in a prospective manner the symptoms and quality of life of those patients having surgery, as compared with patients having balloon dilation (see below), patients having medical therapy with a smooth muscle relaxant (see pages 114 and below), and patients treated with "watchful waiting" (see below)., It is my belief, and the belief of virtually every colleague with whom I have spoken, that there is absolutely nothing inherently risky in a transurethral operation that could result in an increased mortality several years after surgery when compared with the mortality found in a similar group of patients who underwent "open" prostatectomy. Until and unless the evidence from either or both of these studies refutes my belief, I will personally continue to recommend transurethral surgery as the "gold standard" for the treatment of BPH, and I will opt for this procedure myself when it becomes necessary.

Nonsurgical Treatment of BPH. The method of treatment that has gotten the biggest splash in the lay press and that has also achieved some degree of popularity amongst urologists is *balloon dilatation* of the prostate. With this procedure, which can be done on an extremely cost-effective outpatient basis, a balloon catheter is inserted through the urethra and into the bladder and positioned so that the distensible balloon portion of the catheter is within the prostatic urethra (Fig. 9–2). This can be done under fluoroscopic control with the patient sedated and with a local anesthesia inserted into the urethra. In some cases, a general or a spinal anesthesia may be used. Once it has been properly positioned within the prostatic portion of the urethra, the balloon is dilated and this dilation generates a powerful outward force against the prostate gland because the balloon has virtually no "give" to it. These balloons are very similar to those used for balloon dilation of the coronary arteries, although the balloon used for prostatic dilatation is of course considerably larger.

Alternatively, the balloon catheter can be properly positioned in the prostatic urethra either by using direct observation with a cystoscope or by palpating a "button" on the dilating catheter using a finger in the patient's rectum. With any of these methods of placement of the dilating catheter,

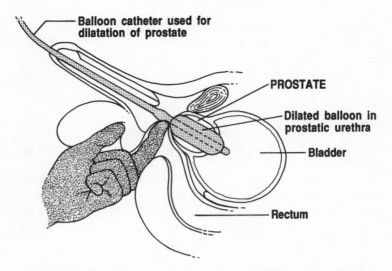

Figure 9–2   *Balloon dilatation of the prostate. Note the inflated balloon within the prostatic urethra and bladder neck. The illustration shows the balloon being properly positioned by the examiner's finger in the patient's rectum where it is palpating a "button" on the dilating catheter thereby ensuring the correct position of the catheter.*

the balloon is then inflated to a diameter of about 2–2.5 cms and this inflation with its great resulting pressure is maintained on the prostate for about ten minutes after which the balloon is deflated and withdrawn. A regular (Foley) catheter (see Fig. 2–9C) is then inserted into the bladder, and it is left in place for two or three days because there is invariably a modest amount of bleeding following this procedure. Patients are often able to return to their normal occupation on the day following the procedure, although not infrequently with a catheter remaining in place for another couple of days.

More than 3000 patients in this country have had balloon dilatation of the prostate to date, and the success of this procedure appears to vary with the enthusiasm of the individual reporting it. Undoubtedly, balloon dilatation in properly selected patients will afford considerable relief of symptoms in half or three-quarters of the patients in whom the procedure is done. However, objective measurements of improvements following balloon dilatation such as voiding flow rate and residual urine usually do not show nearly as much improvement, and the duration of improvement in many patients is often no longer than 2–3 years. It is generally agreed that this procedure should be limited to those patients with a relatively small prostate gland and only minimal enlargement of the median lobe, and it is also generally recognized that any salutary benefits realized from this procedure will probably not be very long-term. How long any beneficial effects of the dilatation will last for any given patient remains to be seen, but certainly the degree and the duration of these benefits as well as any complications of this procedure must be weighed against the proven and long-term benefits of the "gold standard," which is a properly performed TUR of the prostate.

There are some patients who opt for balloon dilatation instead of TURP because they feel that they do not want to risk a resulting retrograde ejaculation following TURP. I must point out to such patients that retrograde ejaculation following balloon dilatation *does* occur if the bladder neck is dilated and this is not infrequently the case. Certainly retrograde ejaculation does not occur nearly as often as it will occur following TURP, but it certainly is not uncommon and you must be aware of this. This procedure is also an extremely attractive option in those patients medically or emotionally unable or unwilling to have a TURP. Although incontinence following balloon dilatation of the prostate is extremely uncommon, I am aware of two cases in which it has occurred in instances in which the procedures were presumably carried out according to standard techniques and guidelines. In summary, I think the enthusiasm for this balloon technique has passed.

Transurethral Incision of the Prostate (TUIP). This is not a recently developed procedure and indeed it has been advocated by some for twenty years or more. However, with the current interest in alternatives to the "gold standard" of TURP, this very simple operation has been of increased interest to some urologists.

Using a resectoscope (see Fig. 6–3) for this operation, the urologist makes deep incisions in the five- and seven-o'clock positions from just inside the bladder neck all the way out to a point just before the external urethral sphincter (Fig. 9–3). That is all—two simple incisions with no attempt to remove any of the obstructing prostate tissue. Those urologists who are enthusiastic about this operative procedure feel that it produces results comparable to that offered by the TURP and that it also has a comparable length of hospital stay and comparable postoperative bleeding. All agree that it is primarily suitable for small prostate glands and undoubtedly its biggest, and perhaps its only, advantage is that it leads to retrograde

Figure 9–3   *Transurethral incision of the prostate. The dotted lines indicate the two positions (five o'clock and seven o'clock) in which deep cuts are made beginning just below the ureteral orifices in the bladder and extending outward to a point just inside the verumontanum. These incisions go all the way through the prostate gland as far as the surgical capsule of the prostate (see page 88).*

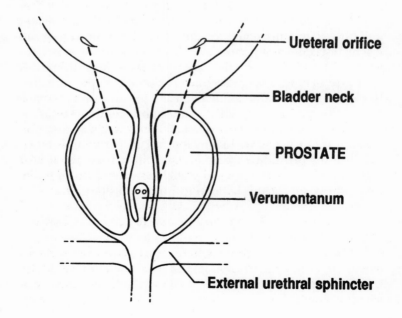

Ureteral orifice

Bladder neck

PROSTATE

Verumontanum

External urethral sphincter

ejaculation much less frequently than TURP. Absent or reduced ejaculation occurs in between 10–25 percent of patients who have this operation; this compared favorably with a 50–70 percent retrograde ejaculation occurrence after TURP, a problem of real concern to some patients.

Since I have had very little experience with this operative procedure, primarily because it appears to have about the same complication rate as the conventional transurethral resection and because the procedure itself has never seemed to me to be as sound, I am unable to recommend it. After all, if you are primarily trying to remove the reasons for an obstruction to the flow of urine, it makes more sense to me to remove the obstructing tissue rather than to simply incise it. For these reasons, I certainly cannot advocate this procedure, but neither would it be appropriate for me to say anything negative about it.

Hyperthermia of the Prostate. There are several different types of equipment currently in use or in various stages of development, and all of these have as their goal the delivery of heat to the prostate gland sufficient to coagulate and then slowly shrink the adenomatous enlargement without damaging the surrounding normal tissue. This heat is delivered at a temperature of 42–55 degrees centigrade by means of a heat-conducting appliance that is placed either into the prostatic portion of the urethra, usually within a urethral catheter, or into the rectum and up against the outside of the prostate gland (see Figure 4–5 to understand the relationship of the rectum to the prostate). The rationale for this type of treatment with hyperthermia has been the observation that increased temperatures applied to the prostate gland have the capability of shrinking the gland and / or shrinking the adenomatous enlargement (the BPH). The differing types of equipment being tested may use different methods of generating the requisite heat.

At least one of these heat-generating microwave machines has already had very extensive use on patients in France (where it was developed) and in England. This rather ingenious machine is referred to as a Prostatron, and clinical trials on an investigational basis have been ongoing at a few centers in the United States since the early part of 1991. These clinical trials are a requisite part of the procedure for any new piece of medical equipment to obtain FDA (Food and Drug Administration) approval before it may be used on a widespread basis.

The heat generated by this machine is conducted through a probe placed within the prostatic urethra; the machine has been engineered so that a cooling fluid applied to the lining of the prostatic urethra limits the degree to which it is heated to about 45 degrees centigrade while the deeper portions of the prostate gland are heated to approximately 55 degrees centigrade. The lower temperature does not result in any significant changes in the tissue heated, but the higher temperature serves to congeal the deeper portions of the prostate gland which results in shrinkage of this tissue within a few weeks' time. By not damaging the lining of the prostatic urethra, the problems of bladder neck contracture and retrograde ejaculation should be obviated. The heat is applied one time only for a period of 30–60 minutes, depending upon the size of the prostate gland, and the entire procedure is done under local anesthetic with no hospitalization required.

The machine itself (Fig. 9–4) is extremely costly and runs in the neighborhood of nearly a million dollars. One of the centers in the United States that has been conducting clinical trials has now been able to follow for a full year 150 patients who have had this treatment for their BPH, and the initially promising results have indeed withstood the one-year test of time. At the end of the one-year follow-up period about one-half of these patients had a definite and statistically significant improvement in their maximum voiding flow rates, and there was a reported success rate, taking both subjective and objective symptoms and findings into account, of 77 percent. Overall, 84 percent of the patients followed for one year reported that they were "happy" with the results of the procedure. These figures are certainly no better, and perhaps not quite as good, as the "gold standard" which is the TURP. However, it is important to realize that the Prostatron operation is done on an outpatient basis with only local anesthesia instilled into the urethra and, therefore, with virtually no morbidity. If the long-

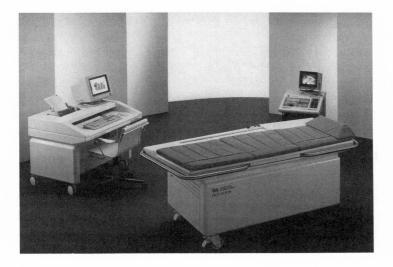

Figure 9–4   *The Prostatron transurethral thermal therapy machine. On the left is the operator's console with computer, keyboard, and printer, and all the necessary software to operate the device. In the center is the patient treatment module in which is housed all the necessary equipment to perform the treatment. On the right is an ultrasound machine that is used to localize the treatment catheter.*

term follow-up (several years) results continue to be as favorable as the one-year follow-up it is certainly likely that the Prostatron may well become the new "gold standard" for relief of bladder outlet obstruction in selected patients. It is doubtful, in my opinion, that it will replace the TURP entirely but it may well earn a place of respect in the treatment of patients with BPH. At present, several university centers in this country and several commercial companies worldwide are trying to develop a hyperthermia device that will be as effective as Prostatron but at a fraction of the cost of Prostatron.

Laser Surgery. This is yet another means of treating benign prostatic hyperplasia; with this modality the laser probe is inserted into the prostatic urethra and prostatic tissue is congealed by means of laser coagulation necrosis. It is now possible to direct the laser beam at right angles to the instrument so that the beam can easily be directed at the obstructing prostate tissue and thus ablate it. Within 2–6 weeks the ablated tissue sloughs out through the urethra. This method appears to have great promise, but its use has been too limited to date for me to attempt to evaluate its long-range efficacy.

The experience of those urologists who have used the laser for ablative surgery on the prostate has been a positive one. The recent addition of the "side-firing" mechanism which works because of a sophisticated quartz prism within the instrument itself has been the real step forward that has made this type of laser surgery much more successful than it had been in the past. Not withstanding this advance and the enthusiasm of those urologists who have worked with the laser for prostate surgery, the method must still be considered as an investigational one that is not as yet in widespread use. It does require a hospitalization, albeit a short one, and it does usually require a spinal or a general anesthetic. There is less blood loss than with a conventional TURP but the long-term benefits and complications are not as yet known. Whether or not it will someday become the "gold standard" remains to be seen. Whether or not it will even compare favorably with the Prostatron also remains to be seen. Certainly, it is all to the benefit of our patients that so many exciting and potentially beneficial alternatives to the current "gold standard" are becoming available, but I believe that we should not in our enthusiasm for the new disregard the old which has achieved such excellent results for so many years.

Transurethral Needle Ablation of the Prostate (TUNA). Perhaps the newest of the "surgical" methods advanced for the treatment of benign prostatic hyperplasia is the transurethral needle ablation of the prostate (TUNA). This procedure is done through the penis under direct vision using a 22Fr. catheter with a fiberoptic system inside it, although it can also be done under ultrasound control using a probe which is placed in the rectum. Using controls on the specially designed catheter, two needles are directed into the substance of the prostate from within the prostatic urethra. These needles are shielded to protect the urethra itself as a radio frequency heats the needles to between 60 and 100 degrees Centigrade resulting in ablation of the surrounding prostatic tissue while avoiding any damage to the urethra itself. The needles are inserted sequentially into various sectors of the prostate until a channel large enough for urine to flow through comfortably has been established. This procedure requires only a local anesthetic and is done on an outpatient basis. As of mid-1993 about 30 patients worldwide have had this procedure, but no trials have begun in the United States; initial trials here are planned for the end of 1993 or early 1994. FDA approval, however, would probably be at least two or three years away. As of now this procedure must be considered an experimental one that may or may not prove to be an acceptable alternative to the "gold standard" TURP. It is estimated that the special equipment necessary for this procedure will cost much less than the special equipment needed for many of the other procedures that might be considered as alternatives to the TURP.

Ultrasonic Aspiration of the Prostate. The use of ultrasound vibrations to disrupt the adenomatous enlargement of the prostate (the benign prostatic hyperplasia) is strictly investigational at this time and its use in patients has been very limited. Through a device very much like a resectoscope, the urologist is able to visually identify the enlarged portion of the prostate and disrupt it by directing the ultrasound vibrations against it. The tissue that is thus disrupted is then aspirated through the resectoscope-like device itself and removed from the patient. A general or a spinal anesthetic is required with this procedure which is done in a hospital on an inpatient basis. The reported advantages of this procedure over the standard form of transurethral resection are a much lower incidence of retrograde ejaculation (which does, however, still occur), less blood loss, and a more complete removal of the enlarged portion of the prostate gland. Whether or not this ultrasound aspiration of the prostate achieves widespread favor remains to be seen, and whether or not it compares favorably with the "gold standard" of transurethral prostate surgery also remains to be seen.

Stents and Coils in the Prostate. Over the past few years various urologists, primarily in Great Britain and the Scandinavian countries, have placed spring-like coiled devices into the prostatic urethra where they are left on either a temporary or semi-permanent basis. More recently, interest in these devices has spread to several centers in this country. These devices serve to stretch the channel within the prostatic urethra thereby aiding the flow of urine. Tolerance of these devices left within the prostatic urethra has been fair with somthing more than half of the patients in whom they have been used reporting a reasonably satisfactory result. Still other urologists have tried placing stainless steel stents within the prostatic urethra using the same rationale as with the coiled devices and with about the same results. Both of these techniques are recommended by their proponents only for palliation in those patients unable to undergo TURP.

Drug Therapy for the Treatment of BPH. On pages 114–15 I mentioned some of the early work and the direction that drug therapy seemed to be taking. In the past 4–5 years many studies have been undertaken, some of which are still ongoing, to fully assess the merit and safety of these various types of medical (nonsurgical and noninvasive) treatment for BPH.

One group of drugs that certainly does have the capability of shrinking an enlarged prostate gland are the *antiandrogens.* These have the effect of reducing circulating testosterone to castrate levels and are able to shrink the prostate in much the same manner that castration will. Unfortunately, these drugs are accompanied by what is generally felt to be a totally unacceptable side effect which consists of loss of libido or erections, or both; hence, these drugs are no longer being used experimentally. Examples of such drugs are estrogens, megesterol acetate, cyproterone acetate, and LH-RH analogs, all of which are, however, used quite successfully in the treatment of prostate cancer (see page 145–46). Also studied in this group of antiandrogens has been eulexin (Flutamide) which does not lead to impotence, but does bring about pain, swelling, and tenderness of the male breast because the increased levels of circulating testosterone resulting from its use are converted by the body to estradiol, an estrogen-related substance that has this effect on the male breast. Flutamide also not infrequently produces nausea, vomiting, and diarrhea and may at times interfere with normal liver function. Flutamide does, however, result in a degree of prostate shrinkage and improvement in voiding symptoms because it prevents the circulating testosterone from binding to the prostate gland itself, and it is this incorporation of the testosterone (and the related dihydrotestosterone) into the prostate that is essential for the maintenance and growth of BPH. Because the testosterone is kept from binding to the prostate, an excess of circulating testosterone results and is converted to estradiol with its resulting unpleasant effect on the male breast.

One very notable exception to the antiandrogen group of drugs that *does* appear to have had a modest success in relieving the symptoms of BPH without any of the unpleasant side effects noted above has been the 5-alpha reductase inhibitor known as finasteride (Proscar). 5-alpha reductase is the enzyme that converts testosterone to the more active dihydrotestosterone, and this latter compound is felt to be largely responsible for the growth of BPH. This drug, Proscar, blocks the action of the 5-alpha reductase and thereby prevents the conversion of testosterone to dihydrotestosterone. It does not, however, appear to have the same negative effects on the male breast or on the gastrointestinal tract as Flutamide. The net effect of using Proscar is that the patient's circulating testosterone remains high but the dihydrotestosterone level is decreased to virtually zero. This results in the salutary effect of causing a modest degree of shrinkage of the enlarged prostate gland without producing any of the widespread unpleasant sexual side effects such as loss of libido or loss of erection.

About 70 centers worldwide, including about 25 centers in the United States, have participated in the evaluation of this drug and these studies were pretty well completed by the end of 1990. Results of this multicenter study were encouraging and about one-third of all of the patients receiving

Proscar demonstrated a shrinkage of the prostate gland with some improvement in the flow of urine. One reason that more patients were not improved may be that BPH (and the normal prostate gland as well—see page 22) is made up of glandular, fibrous, and muscular tissue, and the dihydrotestosterone affects only the glandular portion of the prostatic enlargement. Blocking the formation of dihydrotestosterone would therefore only shrink that portion of the prostate gland enlargement that is made up of prostate glands and would not affect the fibrous and muscular elements of the prostate which may well be more predominant in some men than in others. It is possible that the use of Proscar in younger men with early BPH may prove even more beneficial than in patients with fully developed BPH; these trials are in the initial stages now. It is also possible that regression of prostate size and symptoms will be maximized if Proscar is combined with a smooth muscle relaxant (see below); these trials also are underway.

The long-term side effects of Proscar, if any, are of course unknown, but it does appear that it represents a viable alternative for those patients in whom it works and who are medically unable, or unwilling, to undergo surgery. You should bear in mind that this treatment, as with any of the "medical" treatments mentioned here, requires taking daily oral medications forever. Cessation of the oral medications results in growth of the prostate and the return of symptoms. Use of the drug was approved by the FDA in 1992. Several pharmaceutical companies are actively engaged in research to try to develop new drugs that are chemically related to Finasteride but that might be more efficacious.

Smooth Muscle Relaxants. The action of this class of drugs has already been described on page 114, and in recent years a significant number of patients have participated in trials with this type of drug. Unquestionably, drugs such as prazosin hydrochloride (Minipress) will be beneficial for certain patients in relieving the symptoms of prostatic obstruction and in actually allowing for an improvement in the urinary flow rate. There are longer-acting smooth muscle relaxants, such as ter-

azosin (Hytrin) which has FDA approval as an anti-hyperten-
sion drug but not as an anti-BPH drug. Approval, however,
is tentatively planned for the end of 1993. These smooth muscle
relaxants have their greatest effect on the muscle and fibrous
tissue of the prostate gland rather than the glandular parts of
the prostate which are most affected by the anti-androgen
agents. A combination of these two classes of drugs may yet
prove to be the most salutary approach to the drug treatment
of BPH. All of these smooth muscle relaxants can cause a pronounced drop in blood pressure when a patient suddenly sits
or stands up. For this reason, the dosage of these smooth muscle
relaxants must be adjusted cautiously and increased gradually. Terazosin is being used in the study sponsored by the
American Urological Association that is noted above as one
of the alternative choices to transurethral prostatic resection.

Watchful Waiting. As a result of the published papers mentioned above in which the results and complications (including mortality) of transurethral surgery were called into
question, another option that is being promoted for those
patients having *subjective* indications for surgery *only* (see page
112) is a program of watchful waiting. This alternative is also
part of the research protocol that is currently being sponsored by the American Urological Association. This may just
possibly represent the best alternative to transurethral prostate surgery for the patient who is willing to live with his
symptoms and who does *not* have any of the *objective* indications for surgery (page 113).

My feelings have not changed greatly in recent years, and
in 1993 I still believe that for the patient who is a good surgical risk (the vast majority of patients) transurethral resection of the prostate remains very clearly the procedure of choice
in those patients with objective indications for surgery or for
those patients with subjective indications for surgery but who
clearly say that they want relief from their symptoms. For other
patients, however, who for medical or other reasons do not
want to have this surgery, one of the many alternatives noted
above may indeed prove beneficial.

Chapter 5: Cancer of the Prostate

Surgical Treatment

In discussing stages C and D1 prostate cancer (see pages 139–45) I noted that prevailing urologic opinion was that patients with stage D1 were probably not curable and that in cases where surgical exploration was undertaken, most urologists would opt not to proceed with the radical prostatectomy if any pelvic lymph nodes were found to have cancer in them (stage D1). I also mentioned in the earlier edition of this book that whereas I had formerly been of a like mind with those who felt that cancer in the pelvic lymph nodes made the disease inoperable, I no longer subscribed to that concept because of an increasing body of experience developed by a group of very courageous surgeons who dared to challenge the time-honored concept that lymph node disease made the patient inoperable. Now, six years later, I am more firmly convinced than ever, based upon the published results of radical prostatectomy in several hundreds of patients with stage D1 prostate cancer, that treating these patients with radical prostatectomy and simultaneously orchiectomy is indeed the treatment of choice and that the ten-year survival rate for many of these patients so treated approaches the normal life expectancy that these same patients would have had without cancer. I hasten to add, however, that prevailing urologic opinion remains as it was when I first wrote this book, and the majority of urologists honestly feel that prostate cancer is beyond cure once it is in the pelvic lymph nodes. For this reason they would not proceed with a radical prostatectomy once this disease spread has been demonstrated.

In addition to six valuable years of experience with radical prostatectomy and orchiectomy in stage D1 disease, the great jump forward in knowledge in these last few years has been the indication that the determining factor in the long-term survival of these patients with lymph node positive prostate cancer may be the ploidy pattern of the cancer itself (see above). Diploid tumors, although by far the most common ploidy pattern found in *all* stages of prostate cancer, accounts for just over 40 percent of the stage D1 cancers. These diploid cancers are the ones with the best survival statistics and these do indeed approach the normal life expectancy without cancer when treated with radical prostatectomy and orchiectomy (about an 80 percent 10-year survival). Tetraploid tumors account for about 45 percent of the D1 cancers and have a ten-year survival rate of about 50 percent. Aneuploid tumors account for about 14 percent of patients with D1 cancers and these patients also have a ten-year survival rate of about 50 percent. These survival figures for tetraploid and aneuploid tumors are for those patients treated with radical prostatectomy and orchiectomy.

The ploidy pattern of the tumor is determined by a process known as flow cytometry, and this technique requires a piece of cancerous tissue (from the prostate gland) that is much larger than any that can be obtained by the normal biopsy methods. Therefore, the tissue can most readily be obtained from the surgical specimen removed during the course of a radical prostatectomy. Another and still very new technique, known as static cytometry, can indeed determine the ploidy patterns of a given cancer on a much smaller specimen of tissue, but this technique is not as yet widely available. When it is more readily available, it will be possible to determine the ploidy pattern of a prostate cancer from the tissue obtained during a needle biopsy. This knowledge might perhaps be factored into the decision as to whether or not to proceed with a radical prostatectomy if lymph nodes positive for cancer are found at surgery. I do believe, however, that ten-year survival as well as quality of life survival is better follow-radical prostatectomy and orchiectomy, regardless of the ploidy pattern of the tumor than it is following any other type of therapy or no therapy at all.

Hormonal Treatment

In the treatment of stage D1 prostate cancer (pages 145–48) for those patients in whom radical prostatectomy with examination of the lymph nodes is not performed for whatever reason, or in those patients where spread of the cancer is known to have gone beyond the bony pelvis, i.e to bones or to lungs (stage D2), the treatment of choice remains hormonal. For those patients declining to have an orchiectomy—still the "gold standard"—monthly injections of a long-acting LH-RH analog are available and have been in common use since this book was written. There are at least two companies manufacturing this type of therapy, which is marketed under the trade names of Lupron Depot and Zoladex. These monthly injections must be given by a physician or a nurse and the cost of these medications (exclusive of any charges that may be levied by the physician or the nurse) runs in the neighborhood of something over $3,000–$4,000 per year. One of the problems with this type of therapy is that there is a "flare" of testosterone production in the first week or two after the injections begin. The antiandrogen, Flutamide, acts by inhibiting the binding of testosterone to the prostate and it may be given orally along with the LH-RH analog. This has been found to eliminate the early testosterone "flare" effect and also has been found in some studies to increase overall patient survival by about six or seven months.

Radiation Treatment

Radiation therapy for prostate cancer has already been discussed (pages 136–43 and 178–80) and does indeed remain a viable option for the treatment of prostate cancer that is confined within the prostate gland. However, as I have already noted, I do not feel that radiation therapy alone is of any benefit as far as prolonging life in those patients in whom the cancer has already spread to the lymph nodes. I do believe, though, that radiation therapy combined with orchiectomy is the second best therapy (the best therapy, in my opinion, is total removal of the prostate gland combined with orchiectomy) for these patients with cancer in the lymph nodes. It should be clear, therefore, that before radiation therapy is undertaken, the pelvic lymph nodes should be removed and examined pathologically to determine whether or not cancer has spread to these nodes. This has always involved a formal surgical procedure with its attendant costs, morbidity, and hospitalization, and many physicians (and patients as well) have therefore preferred to carry out the radiation therapy without examining the pelvic lymph nodes.

Within the past couple of years an absolutely remarkable advance in surgical technique, called laparoscopic surgery, has made it possible to remove and examine these lymph nodes without going through a formal and major surgical procedure. This is the same laparoscopic technique that has been popularized recently as a method for removing the gall bladder. Four small incisions, each only about 1 centimeter in size, are made in the lower abdominal wall; the lymph nodes are located and removed by means of very small surgical dissecting instruments that are inserted through three of these holes while a small TV camera with a very bright light source, which has been inserted through the fourth hole, makes it possible for the surgeon to do this dissection and removal of the lymph nodes while watching the TV screen positioned alongside the operating table (Fig. (9–5). Not all centers and not all urologists are using this laparoscopic technique at present, and it is

Figure 9–5   *Operating room setup for laparoscopic surgery. Note the four instruments protruding from the patient's abdominal cavity. Three of these are dissecting and / or grasping instruments and the fourth is a camera with a light source that enables the members of the operating team to view on the TV screen what is being seen and done within the abdominal cavity.*

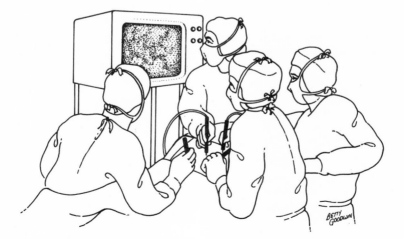

most definitely not applicable in all patients. The hand-eye coordination required of the urologist requires special training followed by hands-on experience. Without a doubt, however, it is something that can readily be done by any urologist who has already undergone the rigors of a formal urology residency training program. You may reasonably wonder whether this laparoscopic technique will ever be applicable to a radical prostatectomy and I would have to say that, for technical reasons, I think it would be extremely difficult, although it may well be on the horizon in the next several years.

Because of this very extraordinary advance in surgical technique, I feel even more strongly at this time that any patient choosing radiation therapy over radical prostatectomy should have removal and examination of his pelvic lymph nodes first in order to spare himself the expense and the discomfort of radiation therapy that is probably not going to help the patient achieve a longer life expectancy.

Radical Prostatectomy via the Perineal Route (Radical Perineal Prostatectomy)

I have been opposed to this surgical approach to the treatment of prostate cancer because it did not allow for sampling of the pelvic lymph nodes through the same incision (see pages 171–75). However, with the present option of removing and examining these lymph nodes by means of the relatively simple and easy (for the patient) laparoscopic approach, the perineal approach to radical prostatectomy now becomes a very viable option. It can be done immediately after the laparoscopic removal and examination of the lymph nodes and it is a perfectly reasonable alternative to the retropubic approach to the prostate (pages 171–75).

Cryoablation of the Prostate

A relatively new and unproven method of treating cancer of the prostate is by freezing it with liquid nitrogen. This experimental procedure is done with the patient asleep (or under spinal anesthetic). Four or five probes are placed through the perineum (the area between the anus and the scrotum) into the prostate gland. Each of these probes is a little larger than 3 millimeters in diameter and they are placed within the prostate by means of ultrasound guidance. Liquid nitrogen is then introduced through these probes into the prostate gland and a little iceball can be seen to form at the end of each probe as it is viewed on the ultrasound screen. Proponents of this cryoablation method of treating prostate cancer feel that this freezing effectively destroys the prostate and the cancer that is within it. It is conceivable that this may indeed be the case but in my opinion this method of treating prostate cancer is experimental and unproven. There are no long-term studies to document the efficacy of this treatment and there are no studies to document that those portions of the cancer that are frozen are actually killed. Moreover, there has not been any proof that all of the cancer present in the prostate is frozen at the time of the procedure since the boundaries of the "killing zone" caused by the freezing are not known. This method of treatment is certainly not without complications even though its advocates say that they are few and far between. Since the boundaries of the tissue destruction are difficult to determine with any degree of certainty, damage to the rectum, which is very close to the prostate (see Fig. 6–7) is not only possible but actually has occurred with resulting fistulous connections between the prostatic urethra and the rectum. This very serious complication results in fecal matter contaminating and infecting the urinary tract and often requires a temporary colostomy until the fistula heals. It is my opinion that this method of treatment for prostatic cancer must be considered experimental. It is one which I cannot recommend because of its unknown and unpredictable success rate. I feel strongly about this because cancer of the prostate has an excellent and well-proven method of treatment in radical prostatectomy and I feel that it is extremely foolhardy for a patient to forgo such an excellent and proven means of treatment for one which is a complete gamble as to its efficacy. Cryoablation may someday prove its proponents to be correct and it may prove to be the "wave of the future" but this can not be said at this time or for many years to come until it has had at least a ten-year post-treatment follow-up so that it can be compared to the results with radical prostatectomy. It should be pointed out that radiation therapy as well has a proven track record and is therefore to be recommended over cryoablation. At the present time in 1993 the use of cryosurgery in the treatment of various urologic disorders has general FDA approval; however, I must emphasize that the specific use of cryosurgery (or cryoablation) in the treatment of cancer of the prostate does definitely not have FDA approval and it cannot receive such approval until and unless this method of treating prostate cancer undergoes rigid and well-controlled clinical testing with a lengthy enough follow-up period after treatment that a judgment can be made as to the efficacy and the complications of the treatment.

Some centers are advocating cryoablation of the prostate for those patients who have already had radiation treatment for their prostate cancers and in whom the radiation therapy has failed and the cancer has recurred. In these patients cryoablation therapy may well be a worthwhile treatment because there really isn't much else to do that has a proven record of success in these cases. "Salvage prostatectomy"— total removal of the prostate—(see Chapter 6) is sometimes considered in cases of radiation failure; it indeed may have merit but the complication rate, particularly incontinence, is high.

Chapter 8: Complications of Prostate Surgery

Retrograde Ejaculation. In the earlier edition of this book I wrote about this condition (see page 215) noting that it was present postoperatively in between half and two-thirds of the patients who have had prostatic surgery (regardless of the approach) for BPH. I went on to point out that the feeling during ejaculation was essentially the same as before the surgery and the only difference was that a man with retrograde ejaculation was essentially sterile and could not father a child (although I did point out that in certain circumstances it was possible to recover the semen from the first voided urine postejaculation and to then use this semen for artificial insemination).

To my great surprise a considerable number of patients wrote to tell me that they were extremely upset because of the retrograde ejaculation that resulted following their TURP operation. None of these men were actively interested in fathering children and so it is possible that they did not pay much attention to what their urologist told them before surgery about this postoperative complication. It is also possible that they may not have been told about it at all.

Most of these men said that indeed their urologist had mentioned it to them beforehand but that they either didn't hear it, didn't understand it, or didn't remember it. Very careful questioning of each of these individuals who took the time and effort to get in touch with me about this problem disclosed to my satisfaction that there were two basic reasons for their great distress: one was that they no longer had the *potential* to father a child, and the other was that since nothing came out of the penis during orgasm and ejaculation these men felt that their manhood, or their sexuality, or perhaps their very being had been compromised. I noted (on page 80) that there is "but one giant synapse between a man's genitals and his brain" and this is another example of what I meant by this. I do not disparage this in any way and I may be no different myself, but it remains a fact with which you and your urologist must contend. Every one of the men who were concerned about fatherhood said that they did not have any plans to father a child at that point in time, but the very comforting thought that fatherhood remained a possibility was no longer with them. Some of these men were concerned about divorce, past, present, or future, and the fact that a new wife might want children. Others with perfectly happy marriages felt that much of their innate manhood had been removed when the potential for fatherhood was removed. One man I remember quite well, a lawyer, was in his late fifties and had never married. He had no particular plans to marry and no special female friend at that time, but he nevertheless was extremely upset at the idea that *if* he should meet someone and *if* he should get married and *if* they should want to have children, it would probably not be possible.

Although the normal sensation of orgasm has been reported to me by many men as being much the same with or without retrograde ejaculation, I must also report that this was contested by those men who felt that the sensation of orgasm was definitely *not* the same after a TUR with resulting retrograde ejaculation and indeed it was definitely not as pleasurable. Some of these men said that although they realized that the surgery they had was medically necessary, they wished in retrospect that there had been some alternative procedure that they might have undergone that would have preserved their normal ejaculatory function.

If you who are contemplating prostate surgery have serious concerns about the foregoing, I think that you should consider some alternative form of treatment for your BPH. Whether it is balloon dilation of the prostatic urethra, transurethral incision of the bladder neck, hyperthermia, or one of the medication treatments, you and your urologist should definitely explore alternative forms of treatment. Although retrograde ejaculation most definitely does occur with balloon dilatation and transurethral incision of the prostate, it is much less likely to occur than with TURP. Will retrograde ejaculation also be a problem with hyperthermia, laser treatment, or drug therapy of BPH? Probably on rare occasion, but not nearly as often as with any of the other methods of treating BPH. If retrograde ejaculation really concerns you—for whatever reason—then you may want to give the most consideration to a regime of "watchful waiting" *if* you do *not* have one of the objective indications for relief of your BPH (see page 113). This occurrence of retrograde ejaculation, I have learned from those of you who have written to me, can indeed be of major concern to some men.

Other Sexual Problems. I had discussed these difficulties in the earlier edition of this book (see pages 212–15) and I thought that I had covered most such problems. However, a few readers have been in touch with me to advise me that my seemingly cavalier attitude about postoperative sexual problems was not justified and that they indeed did have problems that caused them a considerable degree of grief and distress. Some patients told me that although the fact of retrograde ejaculation did not bother them, they were greatly bothered by the absence of the usual pleasurable sensation of orgasm. The best that I could ascertain was that these people said that the feeling was "just different" and the different feeling "not nearly as good as it was before." Even though I know from experience with many patients over many years that this unhappy situation represents the findings of a very small number of patients, I do feel it important to relate this potential problem to you. One very upset patient's wife wrote a letter to me to say that her husband, since his TURP, took an extraordinarily long time to reach a climax and was not even able to do so on every occasion. I am unable to account for such situations as these, but I certainly do not doubt the accurate descriptions of these situations as told to me by these very troubled patients. I do, however, want to reiterate to you that although these problems obviously can and do occur, the great majority of patients who have prostate surgery do indeed return to the same sexual patterns, practices, feeling, and sensation that they had prior to the surgery (except for the retrograde ejaculation).

One final note about the management of erectile dysfunction (impotence) which may follow surgery or may perhaps exist before surgery. Vacuum-producing devices to assist in achieving an erection have been around for a number of years but have only been well-recognized and well-received by physicians and patients in the past few years. These devices are large, clear, snug-fitting plastic cylinders into which the flaccid penis is inserted. The air is then pumped out of the cylinder manually, and this generally results in an erection. The erection is maintained as needed by placing a tight, constricting band around the base of the penis and removing the plastic cylinder, thereby trapping the blood that is necessary for erection within the penis. This form of treatment for erectile dysfunction is preferred by some men, and it can be considered as an alternative to the penile injections (see pages 214–15) (still not FDA approved) or the penile protheses (see page 215). The cost of these vacuum devices is in the neighborhood of $150–$400.

Post Orchiectomy Complications. Most patients do not usually have any major problems—that is, any problems with feminization such as breast enlargement, voice change, change in bodily hair distribution—following orchiectomy except those already noted (see pages 176–78), although occasional "hot flashes" are reported by some patients. Not uncommonly, however, the hot flashes following orchiectomy can become extremely bothersome and a real problem. This situation is probably very much analogous to the situation complained about by some women upon reaching menopause. The reason for the hot flashes is not clear, nor can it be called totally analogous to the menopause situation because in that case the ovarian production of estrogen drops sharply whereas following orchiectomy it is the testosterone production that drops sharply. Nevertheless, the complaints are similar and can be extremely distressing to patients.

I have found that there are three treatments, any one of which may be successful for a given patient. My first choice is the use of Bellergal-S, one capsule twice a day. If this does not work, medroxy progesterone acetate (Provera) in a dose of 10 milligrams a day may help, and if neither of these is of any benefit, I would suggest that you try Premarin (this is conjugated estrogen) in a dose of 0.3–0.6 milligrams a day. In my experience, the extremely unpleasant hot flashes, which may also be accompanied by profuse sweating, can be helped greatly and often eliminated entirely with one of these forms of treatment.

I do hope that the final thoughts in this chapter in *The Prostate Book* will bring the subject up to date for you and will also help to cover those situations that I neglected to cover in the earlier edition of the book. I want to thank all of you whose written and telephone communications to me have formed the basis for much of this additional material, and I also want to thank all of you who have written to me or spoken with me on the telephone for sharing your concerns and problems. I hope this book has been helpful to you.

Glossary

Accessory sex gland a mass of glandular tissue that plays a peripheral (and not a primary) role in procreation.

Acid phosphatase an enzyme made in the prostate gland.

Acute Reaching a crisis rapidly; having a short and relatively severe course; sharp; poignant.

Acute bacterial prostatitis *see* Prostatitis, bacterial, acute.

Adenoma a benign tumor in which the cells form recognizable glandular structures.

Adenomatous enlargement pertaining to the growth of adenoma.

Alkaline phosphatase an enzyme produced in the liver, the bone, and other structures.

American Board of Urology Organized September 24, 1934, the American Board of Urology was incorporated May 6, 1935, and held its first legal meeting on May 10, 1935. The purpose of the board is to render better service to the public by ascertaining the competency of any physician who is specializing, or who wishes to specialize in the field of urology. It arranges and conducts examinations testing the qualifications of voluntary candidates, issues certificates to accepted candidates duly licensed by law (and also holds the power to revoke certificates), and prepares lists of the urologists whom it has certified.

Anesthesia   a loss of feeling or sensation. Although the term is used for loss of tactile sensibility, it is applied especially to loss of the sensation of pain, as it is induced to permit performance of surgery or other painful procedures.

General   a state of unconsciousness, produced by anesthetic agents, with absence of pain sensation over the entire body and a greater or lesser degree of muscle relaxation.

Local   anesthesia confined to one part of the body.

Spinal   anesthesia produced by injection of a local anesthetic into the subarachnoid space around the spinal cord.

Artificial urinary sphincter   a prosthesis designed to restore continence in an incontinent person by constricting the urethra.

Aspiration   the removal of fluids or gases from a cavity by the application of suction.

Needle   removal of cell samples with suction from a specially designed needle which is attached to a syringe.

Prostatic   removal of cell and / or tissue samples from the prostate gland.

Bacteria   unicellular microorganisms that may be harmful to man and may cause infection or inflammation.

Bacterial localization tests   tests devised to isolate the focus of a bacterial infection in order to appropriately treat the infection. A common test is to determine if there is bacterial infection in the prostate or the urethra.

Bacterial prostatitis   infection in the prostate gland caused by bacteria.

Bacteriuria   the presence of bacteria in the urine.

Benign   not malignant; not recurrent; favorable for recovery.

Benign prostatic hyperplasia (BPH)   the nonmalignant but abnormal multiplication of the number of normal cells in prostatic tissue.

Benign prostatic hypertrophy (BPH)   overgrowth of the prostate due to an increase in size of its constituent cells, as opposed to hyperplasia which is the multiplication of those cells. *See also* Benign prostatic hyperplasia.

Biopsy   the removal and examination, usually microscopic, of tissue from the living body which is performed to establish a precise diagnosis.

Bladder   a sac, such as one serving as a receptacle for a secretion. The term is often used alone to designate the urinary bladder.

Bladder catheterization   passage of a catheter into the urinary bladder.

Bladder neck contracture   an abnormal narrowing of the bladder neck such that urine passage is hindered. Can be a complication of prostate surgery.

Bladder outlet   the first portion of the natural channel through which urine flows when it leaves the bladder.

Bladder outlet obstruction   obstruction of the bladder outlet causing problems with urination and / or the retention of urine in the bladder. *See also* Bladder outlet.

Bladder spasm   a sudden and involuntary contraction of the bladder muscle(s), often attended by pain and interference with bladder function.

Bladder trigone   the most dependent and most sensitive part of the bladder. Located at the base of the bladder near the bladder neck.

Blastic lesion   *see* Lesions, blastic.

Blood urea nitrogen (BUN)   A blood test to measure kidney function.

Bone scans   (shortened form of "scintiscan") a two-dimensional picture representing the gamma rays emitted by a radiosotope concentrated in a specific tissue of the body, in this case the bones.

Bone x-rays   x-rays of the bones.

Bulbous urethra   the portion of the urethra just after the membranous urethra and just before the penile urethra.

Cancer   a cellular tumor, the natural course of which is fatal. Cancer cells, unlike benign tumor cells, exhibit the properties of invasion and metastases.

Carcinoma   a malignant new growth made up of epithelial cells tending to infiltrate the surrounding tissues and giving rise to metastases.

Capsule   the structure in which something is enclosed.

Carcinoma   *see* Cancer, carcinoma.

Catheter   a tubular, flexible, surgical instrument for withdrawing fluids from (or introducing fluids into) a cavity of the body, especially one for introduction into the bladder through the urethra for the withdrawal of urine.

Chlamydia   a family of small spherical-shaped bacterial organisms that commonly cause infection in the urethra.

Chronic bacterial prostatitis   the persistence over a long period of time of bacterial prostatitis (infection).

Compensated bladder   a bladder that empties completely on voiding.

Computed tomography (CT) scanning the imaging technique combining x-rays with computer technology to provide a cross-section image.

Continuous or indwelling catheterization   meaning that the patient has a catheter in place in the bladder for a protracted length of time.

Contracture (bladder neck)   *see* Bladder neck contracture.

Creatinine   a normal metabolic waste product the measurement of which in the blood is used as an excellent parameter of kidney function.

Cystoscope   an instrument used for the examination of the interior of the urinary bladder and urethra.

Cystoscopy   direct visual examination of the urinary tract with a cystoscope.

Cytology   the study of cells: their origin, structure, function, and pathology.

Decompensated bladder   a bladder that does not empty after voiding and in which residual urine remains after voiding.

Detrusor   term for the smooth muscle forming the muscular wall of the urinary bladder. On contraction it serves to expel the urine.

Digital rectal examination (prostate)   examination of the prostate by insertion of the finger into the rectum.

Diverticulum   a pouch or sac branching out from a hollow organ structure such as the bladder.

Dribbling, terminal   an involuntary loss of urine at the conclusion of voiding which occurs in drops or in an unsteady stream.

Ejaculate   the semen expelled in a single ejaculation.

Ejaculatory duct   the tubular passage through which the semen reaches the prostatic urethra during orgasm.

Enucleation   the removal of an organ, a tumor, or another body in such a way that it comes out clean and whole, like a nut from its shell.

Enzyme-linked immuno assay   A type of laboratory test in which an enzyme level is determined using an immunological assay.

Epididymis   an elongated, cordlike structure along the posterior border of the testis which provides storage, transit, and maturation of sperm.

Epididymitis   inflammation of the epididymis.

Epithelium   the covering of internal and external surfaces of the body, including the lining of blood vessels and other small cavities.

Erectile dysfunction   impaired or disordered function of the penis regarding its role in vaginal penetration. Also called impotence.

Estrogen therapy   the use of estrogen in the palliative treatment of prostate cancer.

Excretory urogram (IVP)   *see* X-rays.

external urethral sphincter   the ringlike band of muscle fibers that voluntarily constricts the passage of urine from the bladder to the outside.

False negative   the erroneous result of a test when it is reported as negative, but it is truly positive.

False positive   an erroneous report of a test as positive when it is truly negative.

Family physician   the doctor who cares for the family as a whole, usually treating the family unit where appropriate and making referrals to specialists as indicated.

First-glass urine   the term used to describe the first step in a study of the urine in which three glasses are used in order to determine prostate infection as opposed to bladder or urethral infection.

Flow rate (urine)   the measurement of urine as it is expelled from the bladder at its peak period of movement. If this measurement is lower than normal values, it shows that obstruction might be present.

Foley catheter   a catheter which is placed into the bladder for continuous drainage and which is left in place by means of a balloon which is inflated—within the bladder—with liquid.

Fossa   a hollowed out place.

Frequency   the desire to urinate at close intervals.

Gallium scans   An imaging technique for identifying abscesses.

General anesthesia   *see* Anesthesia, general.

General practitioner   a physician who treats a wide variety of medical problems, usually referring patients to appropriate specialists where indicated.

Gland   an aggregation of cells, specialized to secrete or excrete materials not related to their ordinary metabolic needs; also called glandula.

Grading (prostatic carcinoma)   the assignment of a designator to determine the degree of malignancy, based on its microscopic appearance.

Hematuria   blood in the urine.

Gross hematuria   urine in which blood is visible.

Microhematuria   urine in which blood is present, but can only be seen through microscopic examination.

Hesitancy   delayed initiation of the urinary stream.

Hormonal therapy   manipulation of the disease's natural history and symptoms through the use of hormones.

Hormones,   those which are responsible for the secondary sex characteristics of men.

Hyperplastic (prostate) tissue   *see* Benign prostatic hyperplasia.

Hypertrophy *see* Benign prostatic hypertrophy.

Hytrin (terazosin) A drug used in the treatment of hypertension which is helpful in relieving the symptoms of an enlarged prostate (BPH).

Immuno-assay, *see* Radioimmuno-assay

Impotence the lack of ability of a male to initiate or maintain an erection of his penis that is sufficient for vaginal penetration.

Incontinence the inability to control the voiding of urine.

Overflow the condition wherein the bladder retains urine after each voiding and therefore remains virtually full all or most of the time. The urine then involuntarily escapes from the full bladder by "spilling over."

Stress involuntary discharge of urine when there is an increase in the pressure within the bladder, as in coughing or straining.

Total failure of voluntary control of the sphincters (bladder neck and urethral) with constant or frequent involuntary passage of urine.

Indium scans *see* X-rays.

Indwelling catheterization *see* Continuous or indwelling catheterization.

Infection invasion by pathogenic microorganisms of a bodily part in which conditions are favorable for growth, production of toxins, and resulting injury to tissue.

Inflammation redness, and/or heat, and/or swelling, and/or pain caused by irritation, injury, or infection.

Intermittency An inability to complete voiding and empty the bladder on one single contraction of the bladder. A stopping and starting of the urinary stream.

Intermittent catheterization catheterization, usually by one's self, on a systematic interval schedule in order to be certain that the bladder is emptied of *all* urine.

Internist a physician whose specialty is internal medicine.

Isoenzymes one of two or more chemically distinct but functionally identical forms of an enzyme.

Lateral lobes (prostate) The two paired lobes which often grow into the prostatic urethra and cause the symptoms of BPH.

Lecithin granules the granules found in prostatic secretions. They are decreased in bacterial infection in the prostate.

Lesion a wound or injury.

Blastic refers to the increased density of bone seen on x-rays when there is extensive new bone formation due to cancerous destruction of bone.

Lytic refers to the decreased density of bone seen on x-rays when there has been destruction of bone by cancer.

Leydig cells   the cells within the testis that produce testosterone.

Lobes, prostate   There are five distinct lobes of the prostate: two lateral, a middle, an anterior, and a posterior. Only the two lateral lobes and the middle lobe play a role in BPH.

  Lateral   the paired lobes of the prostate which often contribute to BPH.

  Middle   the commonest cause of the symptoms of BPH, the middle lobe cannot ever be felt on digital rectal examination.

Local Anesthesia   *see* Anesthesia, local.

Lutenizing hormone-releasing hormone (LH-RH)   A hormone which acts on the testis to stimulate testosterone production.

Lymph node   a small mass of tissue in the form of an accumulation of lymphoid tissue. Lymph nodes serve as a defense mechanism for the body by removing bacteria and other toxins. They are also a common site for cancer spread.

Lytic lesions   as seen on x-rays, rarefied areas of bone that have been the site of destruction by cancer cells.

Magnetic resonance imaging (MRI)   similar to CT scanning in that cross-sectional images are obtained, an entirely new methodology for imaging. There is no ionizing radiation to which the patient is exposed and no known hazard to this study. It may eventually replace CT scanning as the most advanced and helpful means of imaging available.

male hormones   the androgen hormones which are the masculinizing hormones consisting of androsterone and testosterone.

Male reproductive system   that part of the male concerned with the production, maturation, and transport of sperm to the outside.

Malignant   tending to become progressively worse and to result in death; having the properties of invasion and metastases as applied to tumors.

Membrane   a thin layer of tissue which covers a surface, lines a cavity, or divides a space.

Membranous urethra   that portion of the male urethra that is within the external urethral sphincter muscle. The membranous urethra is in contact with the prostatic urethra on the bladder side and with the bulbous urethra on the penile side.

Mesodermal   one of the three primary derm layers of the embryo. The trigone of the bladder is derived from mesoderm.

Metastatic cancer   cancer that has spread outside of the confines of the organ or structure in which it arose.

Metastasis   the spread of disease (cancer) from one organ or structure to another or to an area removed from the original site of the cancer.

Middle lobes (prostate)   one of the lobes of the prostate gland, not palpable on digital rectal examination, and the lobe that is most commonly the cause of the symptoms of BPH.

Midstream (second-glass) urine   the urine from the middle of the voided stream with the initial and terminal parts of the stream voided elsewhere. The middle portion of the stream presumably contains urine from the bladder, the ureter, or the kidney but not from any portion of the urethra or the bladder neck.

Needle aspiration of the prostate   *see* Aspiration, needle.

Nocturia being awakened during the night by a desire to void.

Nonbacterial prostatitis   inflammation in the prostrate gland in the absence of any demonstrable bacterial organisms.

Nonspecific urethritis   infection in the posterior urethra caused by any organism except the gonococcus organism.

Occult prostatic carcinoma   a carcinoma of the prostate that is neither suspected nor diagnosed but is discovered serendipitously after prostate surgery for BPH. Also called stage A prostate cancer.

Orchiectomy   the surgical removal of both testes.

Oval fat bodies   bodies found in prostatic secretions. They are increased in bacterial infection of the prostate.

Overflow incontinence   *see* Incontinence.

Peak urine flow rate   the maximum rate of flow, in milliliters per second, that a patient is able to generate.

Penile prosthesis   a synthetic material that is inserted into the corpora cavernosa (spongy bodies) of the penis so as to make the penis rigid enough for vaginal penetration.

Penile (or pendulous) urethra   urethra that is in contact with the bulbous urethra and continues all the way to the urethral meatus.

Perineal   pertaining to the perineum, the area of the body between the scrotum and the anus.

Posterior urethra   that portion of the urethra enclosed within the prostate gland and within the external urethral sphincter. These areas are known as prostatic urethra and the membranous urethra.

Primary care physician   the first doctor to see an individual seeking medical care; the doctor also gives continuing medical care during health and illness. Examples are: internists, pediatricians, family physicians, and obstetrician-gynecologists.

Primary sex gland   a gland necessary for reproduction. In the male, the testis is a primary sex gland.

Proscar (Finasteride)   A recently approved drug for the treatment of benign enlarged prostate (BPH).

Prostate or prostate gland   a gland in the male which surrounds the neck of the bladder and the first portion of the urethra as it leaves the bladder. Its principal function is to produce the majority of the fluid in which spermatozoa travel to the outside. It also provides some of the nutrient material for the spermatozoa during their journey. The prostate is made up of connective tissue, muscle, and glandular tissue; it is the glands that manufacture the prostatic fluid.

Prostatic cancer   cancer arising in the prostate; it almost always arises within the glands that are in the prostate.

Prostate specific antigen (PSA or PA)   a recently identified protein that is manufactured in the prostate gland. It is manufactured by both benign and malignant prostate cells.

Prostate surgery

Perineal   an approach to the prostate through the perineum. This approach can be used for the treatment of BPH.

Radical perineal   an approach to the prostate through the perineum; this approach is used to treat prostate cancer. In this operation, the entire prostate gland is removed.

Radical retropubic   an approach through the lower abdomen and behind the pubic bone that is used to treat prostate cancer. In this operation, the entire prostate gland is removed.

Retropubic   an approach through the lower abdomen and behind the pubic bone that is used for the treatment of BPH. It is sometimes referred to as conservative retropubic prostatectomy.

Suprapubic   an approach through the lower abdomen and through the bladder that is used to surgically treat BPH.

Transurethral   a surgical approach done through the urethra to relieve the symptoms of BPH.

Prostatic adenoma   *see* Adenoma.

Prostatic aspiration   *see* Aspiration.

Prostatic biopsy   *see* Biopsy.

Prostatic fossa   *see* Fossa.

Prostatic massage (prostatic stripping)   a digital rectal procedure whereby the index finger forcefully massages each of the two lacteral lobes of the prostate for the purpose of obtaining secretions from the prostate gland. These secretions come out through the urethra.

Prostatic secretions   the fluid that is manufactured in the prostate gland and obtained by means of prostatic massage.

Prostatic urethra   that portion of the urethra that is enclosed within the prostate gland. It begins at the bladder neck and ends at the external urethral sphincter.

Prostatitis, bacterial, acute an inflammation of the prostate gland due to bacterial infection in which the patient is acutely ill.

Prostatitis, bacterial, chronic an inflammation of the prostate gland due to bacterial infection.

Prostatitis, nonbacterial an inflammation of the prostate gland that is not due to bacterial infection. It is presumably caused by an engorgement or statis of prostatic secretions within the prostate gland.

Prostatodynia pain in the perineal, rectal, or suprapubic area that is attributed to the prostate gland. In this condition the prostate gland is entirely normal.

Prostatostasis engorgement of the prostate gland with prostatic secretions due to irregular or infrequent orgasms and ejaculation. *See also* Prostatitis, nonbacterial.

Prosthesis (penile) a synthetic material that is inserted into the penis to make it rigid enough to allow for vaginal penetration. It is used for patients with erectile dysfunction (impotence).

Proteinuria the presence of protein in the urine. Small amounts of protein in the urine (up to 150–200 mg per 24 hours) are normal, beyond that is considered abnormal.

Pubic symphysis the joint, formed by a union of the bodies of the pubic bones in the midline by a thick mass of fibrous, cartilagenous material. It is the hard area felt by pressing firmly on the pubic hair line.

Pyuria the presence of white blood cells (pus cells) in the urine.

Radical prostatectomy the radical or total removal of the entire prostate gland that is done for the treatment of prostate cancer.

Radio-immuno assay an immunological technique for the measurement of minute quantities of antigen or antibody, hormones, certain drugs and other substances found within the body.

Radioisotope an isotope which is radioactive, thereby giving it the property of decay by one or more of several processes. Radioisotopes have important diagnostic and therapeutic uses in clinical medicine and research.

Rectal examination (prostate) the insertion of an examining finger into the rectum for the purpose of feeling the prostate gland.

Renal scans (renal scanning) the production of a two-dimensional picture (the scan) representing the gamma rays emitted by a radioactive isotope concentrated in a specific tissue of the body, in this case the kidney. Renal scans are used to determine blood flow to the kidney, kidney function, and obstruction to drainage to the kidney.

Resection (transurethral) the removal of obstructing BPH prostate tissue that is done from within the urethra.

Resectoscope the instrument that is used for a transurethral resection.

Residual urine any urine that is left behind in the bladder immediately after voiding. The normal residual urine is zero cc.

Retention (urinary) the inability to void when the bladder is full. This is usually caused by obstruction to the flow of urine from benign prostatic hyperplasia.

Retrograde ejaculation semen going backwards into the bladder, instead of through the urethra to the outside, during orgasm and ejaculation. This is sometimes caused by an incomplete closure of the bladder neck during orgasm and ejaculation which frequently follows transurethral resection of the prostate gland.

Retropubic the area behind and below the pubic bone and pubic symphysis.

Scans (scanning)

    Bone the production of a two-dimensional picture (a scan) representing the gamma rays emitted by a radioactive isotope concentrated in a specific tissue of the body, in this case the bone. When new bone is being laid down in a given area (a reparative phase) there is an increased uptake of the radioisotope in that area. The laying down of new bone may be in response to bone destruction from cancer spread to the bone but it may also be in response to bone trauma or even to arthritis. An increased uptake of a radioisotope in one or more bones of a patient known to have prostatic cancer strongly suggests that the cancer has spread to those bones.

    Renal *see* Renal scans

Scrotum the pouch or sac which contains the testes and their accessory organs.

Second-glass (midstream) urine the urine that is collected from the middle of the voided stream after the initial part of the urinary stream has been discarded and before the terminal part of the stream has been discarded. Collection of only the middle portion of the urinary stream, or the second-glass urine, is a technique for examining the urine from the bladder, ureter, or kidney and for excluding possible bacterial contamination that might come from the urethra or the prostate.

Secretions, prostatic the fluid that is manufactured within the many glands of the prostate gland.

Semen   the thick, whitish secretion of the reproductive organ in the male; it is composed of spermatozoa in their nutrient plasm, secretions from the prostate, seminal vesicles, and various other glands.

Seminal vesicle   a pouch or sac that is a paired structure and located just behind the bladder. It provides nutrient material for the spermatozoa and may store spermatozoa as well. It empties into the prostatic urethra through the ejaculatory duct at the time of orgasm and ejaculation.

Seminferous tubules   the microscopic tubules within the testis where spermatozoa are manufactured.

Sexual dysfunction   a less-than normal functioning of the structures by which reproduction is achieved. An inability to achieve an erection, to maintain an erection, or to ejaculate would all be examples of sexual dysfunction.

Sitz bath   a small amount of water in the bottom of a bathtub that is just sufficient to cover the perineal area when a patient sits in it. When the water is warm and when various bath salts are added to it, it can have a palliative effect on perineal pain or discomfort.

Skinny-needle prostatic aspiration   the new technique by which cells from suspicious areas of the prostate are aspirated for examination. This is a form of biopsy that is becoming increasingly popular and accepted to evaluate abnormal areas of the prostate gland.

Spasm   a sudden, violent, involuntary contraction of a muscle or a group of muscles.

Spermatozoa   the mature male germ cell which is the specific output of the testes. It is the generative element of the semen, which serves to fertilize the ovum.

Sphincter (urinary)   the muscle which a man voluntarily contracts when he wants to shut off his urinary system. It is located just beyond the prostate gland, going towards the penis, and the membranous portion of the urethra is enclosed within it.

Spinal anesthesia   *see* Anesthesia, spinal.

Spongy body   the slang term for the two corpora cavernosa which are the structures within the penis that become engorged with blood during erection. When penile prostheses are used to treat individuals who are unable to achieve an erection, these paired prostheses are placed into the two corpora cavernosa of the penis so as to simulate the actual erectile process.

Staging (prostatic cancer)   the process by which various tests are done to determine whether or not a prostatic cancer is still confined within the prostate gland or has spread outside of it.

Stress incontinence   the inability to control the flow of urine, with resulting involuntary loss of urine, when there is an increase in intra-abdominal pressure such as occurs with sneezing or coughing.

Stricture, urethral   a scarring or narrowing within the urethra that can produce symptoms of voiding difficulty very much like the symptoms of BPH. The stricture or scar within the urethra is often caused by an injury to a specific area within the urethra.

Suprapubic   above or superior to the pubic symphysis and pubic bone. This is the specific term used for the area of the abdomen above the pubic symphysis and the pubic bone and it also refers to one of the surgical approaches for treatment of benign prostatic hyperplasia.

Surgical capsule (prostate)   not a capsule at all but simply the interface between the benign prostatic hyperplasia and the true prostate gland. During surgery for the relief of BPH all of the tissue within or inside this surgical capsule is removed, leaving behind the true prostate tissue.

Testosterone   the principal circulating male hormone.

Therapy

Estrogen   a treatment for androgen-dependent cancer of the prostate. By giving estrogens, the circulating androgen level is effectively reduced to castrate levels. This is one of the types of hormonal types of therapy or hormonal manipulation that is used for the treatment of cancer of the prostate.

Hormonal   a generic term to indicate reduction of the male hormone to castrate levels in the treatment of cancer of the prostate.

Third-glass urine (postprostatic massage)   the urine that is collected immediately following the prostatic massage which contains the secretions from the prostate gland that have pooled in the prostatic urethra. Examination of this third-glass urine following the prostatic massage is necessary in order to differentiate between infection in the urethra and infection in the prostate and also to differentiate between infection and simple inflammation within the prostate gland.

Tissue   a collection of similar specialized cells united in the performance of a particular function.

Trabeculation (of the bladder)   the condition of the bladder muscle when it has undergone a work buildup because of obstruction to the flow of urine from BPH. The buildup of the bladder muscle is irregular and induces a swiss cheese appearance within the bladder consisting of very prominent bands of built-up muscle separated by recessed areas with no apparent buildup of the muscle. The appearance of trabeculation in the bladder is strong evidence of bladder outlet obstruction, usually due to benign prostatic hyperplasia.

Transurethral the route through the urethra. The term usually applies to something being passed into or through the urethra as, for example, a catheter, a cystoscope, or a resectoscope.

Trigone (bladder) the most dependent and most sensitive portion of the bladder at the base of the bladder near the bladder neck.

True capsule (prostate) the fibrous layer of tissue that surrounds the true prostate tissue in much the same manner as the skin of an apple surrounds the pulp of the apple.

Tru-cut biopsy needle the traditional hollow lumen needle which is used to remove a "core" or "plug" of tissue from a solid structure (such as the prostate). It is removed for microscopic examination to determine whether or not cancer is present.

True prostate tissue the substance of the normal prostate gland. It is made up of fibrous or connective tissue, muscle tissue, and glandular tissue.

Ultrasound (ultrasonography) a technique for the visualization of structures deep within the body by recording the echos of ultrasonic waves directed into the tissues. Ultrasonography is a noninvasive imaging technique for detecting masses within the body and for differentiating cystic masses from solid masses. It is also used as an aid in performing biopsies of the prostate.

Uremic poisoning (uremia) the retention and failure to eliminate excessive by-products of protein metabolism in the blood and the toxic condition produced thereby. It is characterized by nausea, vomiting, headache, dizziness, coma, or convulsions and, ultimately, death. The condition is usually caused by kidney failure.

Urethra the canal or channel through which urine is conveyed from the bladder to the exterior of the body. It is divided into anatomic areas beginning at the bladder neck.

Bulbous has the largest diameter of any portion of the urethra. It begins at the end of the membranous urethra and continues to the penile or pendulous portion of the urethra.

Membranous that portion of the urethra contained within the external urethral sphincter. It begins at the end of the prostatic urethra and ends at the beginning of the bulbous urethra.

Penile (or pendulous) that portion of the urethra contained within the penis.

Posterior the term used for the prostatic urethra and the membranous urethra taken together.

Prostatic that portion of the urethra beginning at the bladder neck and ending at the external urethral sphincter. It is contained entirely within the prostate gland.

Urethral stricture an abnormal scar or narrowing at any point within the urethra. It is usually caused by an injury to the urethra.

Urethritis, Nonspecific an infection of the posterior urethra that can be caused by any microorganism except the gonococcus organism.

Urinary sphincter *see* Sphincter, urinary.

Urine analysis the physical, chemical, and microscopic analysis and examination of urine.

Urine culture the incubation of urine at a specific temperature and in a specific media so as to permit the growth and identification of microorganisms. This is the definitive means by which an infection in the urinary tract is diagnosed.

Urodynamic studies quantitative means by which the two principal functions of the bladder, consisting of urine storage and urine evacuation, can be measured.

Urologist a physician who specializes in the medical and surgical treatment of diseases of the urinary tract in males and females and the reproductive tract in males. A urologist must have had at least five years of hospital training following graduation from medical school and must also have passed the written and oral examinations given by the American Board of Urology.

Urothelium the lining of any portion of the urinary tract.

Vas deferens the muscular, tubular structure that propels and transports spermatozoa from the epididymis into the prostatic urethra.

Weak urinary stream a voided stream that has less than normal expulsive force to it. This can be quantitated by measuring the maximum urinary flow rate expressed in milliliters per second.

Work hypertrophy (of the bladder) the muscle buildup that occurs within the bladder in response to the new growth of BPH tissue which makes bladder emptying more difficult. The actual buildup of muscle within the bladder is called trabeculation.

X-rays electromagnetic vibrations of short wavelengths that can penetrate most substances to some extent, thus revealing the presence and position of fractures or foreign bodies. They can also cause some substances to fluoresce, by which the size, shape, and movement of various organs can be observed.

Index